The Health Project Book

The Health Project Book is a practical and detailed guide to all aspects of conducting a research project in health. Neil Wood has supervised student projects in health over many years and this handbook is based on his experience in teaching students how to get the best out of themselves and their project.

Individual chapters cover:

- ethical considerations
- the selection of samples
- questionnaire design
- working in a laboratory
- conducting interviews
- statistical and qualitative analysis.

Case studies illustrate the use of:

- CD-ROM facilities
- the Cochrane database on the world wide web
- qualitative analysis software.

The Health Project Book encourages a systematic approach. It will be an extremely useful resource for students and professionals in nursing, health studies, health sciences, psychology and related fields.

Neil Wood is Co-ordinator of Research and Development, BHB Community Health Care NHS Trust, Essex, UK.

Contents

Figures and Tables

Figures

Tables

Preface

It is common practice for students on health-related courses to undertake a piece of supervised research as part of their degree programme. This book is written for such students who may be undertaking a project which involves either the collection of numerical data or data suitable for qualitative analysis. It is therefore a practical guide to a range of research techniques which are commonly used in student projects, although I have tried to avoid a 'cook book' approach, so that the need to understand the strengths and limitations of various research approaches is emphasised. This book has derived from handbooks that I have written for my own students on the BSc(Hons) degree in Health Studies at University College Chichester, who have tackled a wide range of projects including work in alternative medicine and immunology and more traditional areas of nursing, psychological or sociological research. The material in the book should prove of particular value to those who may have forgotten much of what they learned on research methods courses. It should be helpful to such students on health studies, nursing, psychology, sports science and pre-clinical medical courses. The book may also prove of some value to postgraduate students in these and related disciplines to accompany a course on research methods.

It is usual even in introductory books on statistics and research methods for authors to provide statistical formulae and computational techniques for working out the formulae. I have avoided this approach, as it is my experience that many students generally find these of little relevance nowadays when computers are routinely used to run analyses. There are plenty of statistics textbooks for those who need this information; I have been concerned instead to convey some appreciation of the decisions and assumptions behind the commonly used statistical analyses. Similarly, it is outside the remit of this handbook comprehensively to discuss the many differing standpoints and debates associated with qualitative analysis; these can appear remote and theoretical when the immediate need in a student project is typically to produce an analysis of interview transcripts or similar material. I have tried to emphasise a systematic approach to this, and generally throughout the book; Chapter 11 provides an example of the use of a computer software package to accomplish the task. This book is certainly no substitute, therefore, for the reading of specialist texts on research design, statistical or qualitative methods, but should provide a handy starting point for the aspiring health researcher in each of these areas as well as on a number of other topics not routinely covered in methods textbooks, such as the use of the internet.

Neil Wood
March, 2000

Acknowledgements

This book derives from course material I prepared for BSc(Hons) Health Studies students at University College Chichester. Any book, and especially an introductory text such as this, inevitably draws widely upon ideas and material which derive from others, even though all influences many not be explicitly acknowledged or even recognised. In preparing this volume, I am particularly indebted to Dr Peter Green for the interview material he kindly provided and which is introduced in Chapters 10 and 11. I am also grateful to colleagues who read and commented upon drafts of this volume including Beverley Hale, Elizabeth Kemp, Gill Kester, Anand Kumar and Sue Rowley from University College Chichester, Trudi James from Southbank University, Martin Orrell from University College London and John Sitzia from Worthing Priority Care NHS Trust. They have helped to shape the direction and content of the final book, whilst any errors and inaccuracies of course remain my own. Last but not least, I extend a warm 'thank you' to my family for putting up with many hours of my unsociability when I was researching and writing this volume. To these, and many others I have failed to mention by name who have helped me along the way, my grateful thanks.

Chapter 1

Before you start

Getting going

Welcome to the world of research! A student research project is an opportunity to apply all the 'real world' skills which degree programmes aim to impart. Overall, your project should reflect your ability to sustain an in-depth enquiry on a health-related topic. The broad field of health-related research includes topics which may explore largely psychological, social, biological, medical or nursing issues, and examples in these fields are chosen throughout this volume.

As the first stage of beginning to plan your project, you need to think about what is practical to achieve as opposed to what is ideal or desirable. Thus you have an ultimate deadline by which to complete and write up your project report. You may also be limited by the availability of practical resources such as specialised facilities. A frequent constraint arises through the need to gain access to certain client or patient groups for some investigations and, if the idea you have in mind involves access to such individuals, you need to check in advance that the necessary permission is obtainable. You may decide to conduct a study because there is particular expertise, in the form of supervision and a research tradition in your department, in a particular field, and such support can be invaluable. Your tutors may suggest a project is carried out within particular areas, although the precise way in which it is conducted may be open to discussion and negotiation.

The planning stage is perhaps the most crucial stage in the conduct of any piece of research. Research which is entered into where the aims are woolly and ill-defined on the assumption that 'things will work out in practice' is almost certainly doomed to failure. The process of deciding upon a suitable research question and how to go about addressing it should not be rushed. You may have a few general ideas within some areas of inquiry and may need to hone your ideas by consulting literature in the library or conducting some CD-ROM or internet searches. You need to get an early 'feel' for what is known about the subject you have in mind and whether previous research has come up with definite conclusions. You will probably also want to bounce your ideas off friends, colleagues or members of academic staff before finally deciding on your particular research question. Alongside this process of deciding on your research question, you need to be thinking about the techniques and methods that you might employ in order adequately to address it.

The processes that you may employ in order to assist the planning of your research are as many and varied as there are researchers. Some people find that they like to sit down with a large sheet of paper and make a visual representation of the overall structure of the project, perhaps in the form of a flow diagram with arrows and boxes representing various stages of the data collection process. Others may find that the use of a project management package on a personal computer can be helpful to identify critical stages and intermediate goals to be achieved by certain dates so that the project can be completed on time. An example chart of the output from such software is shown in Chapter 14 of this book. Yet others find a more unstructured approach to be helpful. For instance, most word processors have an outliner which allows you to set up in a hierarchical manner headings and sub-headings under which ideas about the project can be filled in as they come to you.

Whatever method is adopted, you will find it much easier if you are organised! So develop a system for keeping track of your references from the earliest stage. A haphazard pile of reprints and hastily scribbled notes are unlikely to provide the degree of organisation you will need. Typing referencing information about relevant papers, together with a summary of what they are about, into a database on a personal computer is a much more systematic approach. An equivalent goal can be reached by the use of a simple card index system; cards can then be sorted in order of topic or author. Your database of relevant literature will grow and evolve over the course of your study as more work is identified of relevance to your research, and you should be thinking about the implications of it all for your own project.

The overall general stages involved in planning, implementing and reporting a research study are illustrated in Figure 1.1. Although this is the general sequence of steps involved, it should be borne in mind that the process is not always such a linear and sequential one. For example, although the background literature searching in most studies should come at an early stage when the study is being planned, this may continue throughout the project. Data collection, analysis and interpretation sometimes proceed hand in hand, especially in qualitative research studies as is discussed in Chapters 10 and 11.

In planning the timescale of your project, you should allow a contingency element for slippage at all critical stages of your investigation. One of the key distinguishing features of successful planning of a research project is the ability to anticipate, as far as possible, potential difficulties which may arise along the way and to make contingency plans in the event of them arising. Critical pieces of laboratory equipment can fail, and may take weeks or months to be repaired. Or permission may suddenly be withdrawn by an organisation once a study has commenced in response to ongoing events. It is normal for some research subjects to fail to keep appointments or for people to forget to do things. The way that you handle the research problems will be an indicator of the quality of your research and of your initial planning to meet such contingencies.

The outcome of any non-trivial piece of research is never certain, otherwise there would be little point in carrying out the work. However, some investigations are more risky than others in the likelihood of generating usable data. In particular, it is vital that the methods of data collection and analysis that you have selected must be capable, *in principle*, of answering the questions originally posed, even if in the event the study was inconclusive. A study which cannot reasonably be expected to provide an answer, even in principle, to the questions you have set in your aims and objectives is going to fail.

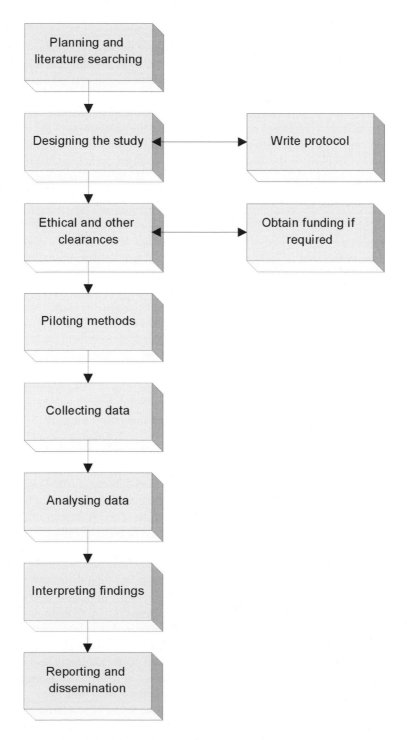

Figure 1.1 Steps involved in a research study from initial idea to conclusion

The research process

It is a main aim of this book to encourage a well thought out project conducted to high standards of research inquiry. Although my background is rooted within the scientific research tradition, some researchers within the very broad field of health-related research would not necessarily agree with their work being labelled as 'scientific'. Enthusiasts of 'post-positivistic' or 'new paradigm' research tend to downplay measures taken to increase objectivity, which are viewed as being at the expense of the naturalness of the setting and of an intuitive and empathetic approach to the understanding of the world of people. This issue is taken further in this book on the discussion of qualitative approaches in Chapter 10; the broad field of health research has been enriched by a great diversity and variety of research approaches and methods. Whatever our philosophical and emotional leanings in the field of health, however, it is important that researchers demonstrate an underlying integrity in their enquiries.

People often carry out a piece of research because they have perhaps a passionate, or personal, interest in the area of inquiry – whether this is gender discrimination, the effect of budget cuts on patient care or treatment for alcoholism. These sincerely held personal convictions and values are not, by themselves, reasons for not conducting research within the field, and indeed motivate much work which appears in the scientific literature. Nevertheless, it is danger to seize upon a project as an opportunity to 'prove a point' and attempt to present the results in such a way as to influence existing systems in desired directions. It is usually obvious to any disinterested reader when this has been done, and this approach is therefore, apart from being scientifically unethical or dishonest, also ultimately self-defeating. Policy indications may, of course, flow from findings in due course, and if these are recognised by the researcher they should be included in the discussion – but they will only be valid if an unbiased stance has been taken towards the collection and analysis of the data.

Where research integrity is compromised, research treads a dangerous path. Some of the worst excesses have been committed by researchers, once regarded as eminent, whom we now know to have systematically distorted, and even fabricated, their research data for ideological ends. The history of the development of IQ tests and their subsequent application in the early and middle years of the twentieth century to 'prove' the genetic inferiority of black and working class people is a sorry and salutary tale for any researcher. Research of course is never neutral or 'value free'; it is, after all, conducted by human beings with particular values and attitudes and is carried out within the context of a social structure where individuals have particular roles and responsibilities. Society, in the form of established structures, will ultimately set the agenda for research – either directly, for example, through the funding of research or more subtly through the questions and paradigms, or systems of beliefs, that it will support.

Books on research often include some brief – and occasionally thought provoking – 'philosophy' written for the benefit of the aspiring researcher, which is designed to get you thinking critically about the process and context as much as the outcomes and specific methods of your research. So here goes! The notion of the 'gradual accumulation of knowledge towards the truth' is generally not how research proceeds. Rather, it is normally a case of blind alleys and false trails, and sometimes of going completely in the wrong direction.

The currently accepted 'pot' of knowledge in any one social or scientific discipline can be likened to a pot of coins; some coins in the pot will be bright and shiny, and these represent carefully designed, well conducted studies producing reliable data. These will mingle with many others which are tarnished to one degree or another through bias, ideological distortion on the part of the researcher, or simply bad design. The journal peer review refereeing system – whereby research papers are sent out by journal editors to fellow researchers in the field for comment – will generally weed out the worst excesses, so that hopefully most of the bent coins will never even get thrown in. However, research is a democratic process where all shapes and sizes of coin, and different currencies, are thrown into the pot and made available to the research community.

Sometimes the odd bad penny will be shown to be a forgery and will be ejected. Most of the time, however, the bad stays in, confusing the picture until it becomes recognised only very slowly. As research directions change, better theories emerge and previous papers fail to be cited in the literature. Unfortunately, the abilities of those who are picking up the coins – the other research workers and society generally – are impaired, and it is difficult to distinguish the shiny from the dull. Some will have the insight, as well as the necessary resources in the form of research grants, to conduct large studies or buy the electron microscopes, the laboratory equipment and so on to improve their discrimination and will be generally ahead in their thinking. Many others will have to accept, or be content to accept, what others tell them about the contents of the pot.

Very occasionally a gold coin – a real conceptual advance in a field – will be so shiny that it will stand out to most people, although not necessarily at first. A minority of sceptics will argue that it is false gold, and sometimes history will prove them right. Once in a blue moon, the whole pot is knocked over and a different vessel of a new shape and size has to be started again. So a Darwin or an Einstein will come along and Newton's classical mechanics is supplanted by Einstein's relativity theory, providing a major new paradigm wherein it becomes necessary to ask completely different sets of questions. These qualitative shifts in the mindset and world view of scientists have been described as 'scientific revolutions' by the philosopher of science, Thomas Kuhn.

A worthwhile contribution to this fund of knowledge or ideas should be the aim of a good research study, even if the particular objectives of a study are quite limited and practical. To achieve this, perhaps the over-riding factor to guard against by the conscientious investigator is bias. There are many sources of potential bias which can affect a research project at any level; some are inherent in the way studies are designed, some by the way studies are conducted. This book aims to point up such potential distorting influences and ways of guarding against them. For example, experiments are often conducted 'blind' – that is, without knowledge of which people have been allocated to which group in order to minimise the effects of experimenter expectations on the outcome, a form of bias which has been called the Rosenthal effect. Other techniques which are used by researchers to minimise bias, or systematic error, in their methods and approach are specifically discussed in Chapter 3 which introduces different ways of collecting data; Chapter 4 discusses issues concerned with sampling, Chapter 5 concentrates upon questionnaire design techniques, Chapter 6 discusses the experimental method and Chapters 10 and 11 are devoted to a discussion of qualitative approaches. All researchers within the field of health, whatever their method of approach, need to be aware from the start of potential ethical issues involved in their projects and the next chapter introduces some of these.

Action points

- Start your collection of references and other material as soon as possible.
- Explore the feasibility of the techniques you have in mind.
- Consider the strengths and weaknesses of alternative research designs.
- Plan out your approach.

Chapter 2

Matters ethical and otherwise

Virtually all research raises some questions of ethical interest. It is not only researchers at the 'leading edge', where animal or human experimentation is concerned, who need to be acutely aware of the ethical implications of what they are contemplating. An apparently innocuous questionnaire survey may have considerable ethical ramifications, for instance on the attitudes or psychological state of those taking part, depending on how and why it is being administered and used. The identification and selection of appropriate individuals in a sample is subject to ethical considerations. Likewise, the reporting of research results demands high ethical standards and integrity from the researchers.

Some projects may involve the use of patients or clients selected, for example, from hospital or GP lists or may involve conducting work using NHS premises or facilities. Appropriate local research ethics committee clearance needs to be obtained in advance for any such project work, even if the contact with the patients or ex-patients involves no more than the sending out of a letter or questionnaire. Many such committees only meet occasionally and it is important to submit an ethical committee application well in advance of the planned start date for data collection.

Although ethical committee procedures differ, depending upon the health authority, you are likely to be sent a lengthy form to complete. This will require information concerning, for example:

- qualifications and function of people involved in the project
- objectives of the study
- scientific background to the research
- design of the study
- information on potential benefits and risks of the work
- how research subjects will be recruited
- how informed consent will be achieved
- precautions taken to protect confidentiality
- copies of information sheets, consent forms and questionnaires.

Prior to ethical committee approval being obtained, it is, of course, permissible to carry out some preliminary work on the project such as the devising of questionnaires and literature searching, but you need to bear in mind that some people find their proposals rejected by an ethics committee and you may have seriously to rethink your approach once the project is under way. It cannot therefore be emphasised enough that if your proposed research needs to go to a hospital ethics committee that you write to the chair of the committee well in advance of the proposed start date of your project, outlining what you intend to do and obtaining dates by which applications have to be submitted. Some ethics committees do not meet regularly and, if you miss a deadline for submission, your project may be held up for several months.

One way to avoid the need to obtain local research ethics committee permission with a client group is to obtain a viable sample through a method which does not involve access to NHS patient lists. For example, research subjects in some instances may be contacted through an informal local support group. If the group facilitator or organiser, as well as each individual contacted, provides personal permission and volunteers to help with the study, such a study need not go before a hospital ethics committee, although you may need to submit the study to scrutiny from a local university or other appropriate ethics panel.

Information which personally identifies individuals must not be entered onto a computer without application and registration with the Data Protection Registrar, which is costly and impractical for student projects. This is a legal requirement governed by the Data Protection Act, 1984. If names and addresses, or even postcodes, are collected, these must not be entered onto the computer along with the data collected. In most student projects, it is safer not to record such identifying information, or to ask for it, unless in exceptional circumstances – for instance, if individuals need to be contacted again for follow-up at a later stage.

If research subjects are being obtained through clubs, societies or similar, before any approach is made to individuals, an initial approach should be made to the manager or person in charge and the proposed project discussed and approval obtained in principle. If this is obtained, permission may also be needed from other individuals such as line or area managers. This permission should be obtained in writing. Draw up a short letter and obtain the signatures of the relevant individuals so that copies of these can be included in an appendix to your project report, so there can be no dispute afterwards over the nature of the permission which was obtained.

Written consent must also be sought from the participating research subjects on an individual basis, including consent to conduct an interview or obtain information from stored records. In the case of people under 18 years old, consent must also be obtained from a parent or guardian. On consent forms, confirmation is required of each subject that:

- the volunteer is willing to take part in the study
- the researcher has explained the nature and purpose of the study and has informed the subject of any risk that the researcher foresees
- the subject has received information about the essential features of the study, including information in respect of attendances at research sessions
- the subject has been given an opportunity to question the researcher and has understood the researcher's advice
- the subject has been told s/he is free to withdraw consent at any time without the need to justify the decision.

An example of an information sheet and a consent form, which were approved by a local ethics committee, is shown on pp. 9–10. These were prepared for a study concerned with evaluating a child health service which involved conducting interviews with parents, children and staff involved in providing the service.

Assessment of the Integrated Child Health Service
Information for those taking part

Why is this study being done?

In 1997 the services for children in this area were reorganised to try to improve the way health care and help is given to local children and their families.

To make sure that the changes are the right ones for improving the services, we need to ask for your views on a number of issues.

We are asking a range of people to take part who are interested in making sure children get as good a deal as possible from the service. This includes doctors, nurses, therapists, health visitors, managers, parents and children, as well as the health authority itself.

What will my involvement be?

All we are asking of you is about an hour of your time to answer some simple questions relating to the service.

Families

We value the comments from both parents and children. If your child (who is receiving care from the service) would like to take part and you happy for this to happen, the researcher will be pleased to arrange for you each to talk about the service from your own points of view.

Who will know what answers I gave?

Only the researcher who interviews you will be able to identify who you are, the information you give will not have any of your personal details kept with it. Some of the comments people make might be used to help explain an issue when we share the overall results of the work. None of these comments will be identified with the person who made them unless we ask specifically for their permission (and you are happy to give it) before using them. Nothing you say during the interview will be shared with anyone else except in such a way that they will not be able to identify you, without obtaining your permission first.

What if I choose not to take part?

It is hoped that all those employed by the service will have no objection to being interviewed, although we respect that everyone has a right to refuse should they so wish, without affecting their work in any way.

Parents and children also have the right to refuse and in all cases, deciding not to take part will not make any difference to the care your child (and you) receives in any way.

Thank you very much for reading this information leaflet. If you have any further questions or concerns about this evaluation, you can contact: *(contact details provided here)*

Staff / Parent Consent Form

I have had this evaluation explained to me and received a copy of the information leaflet.

I agree to being interviewed by the researcher as described in the leaflet and am happy for comments I make to be used providing they are not identified with me.

I understand that I am free to stop being involved in the evaluation at any time without affecting the care my child receives (if he or she is a patient) or my job (if I am a member of staff).

Signed. . . . .

Name . . . .

Address . . . .

. . . .

. . . .

Witnessed by . . . .

Researcher . . . .

Children's consent form

I would like to take part in this project looking at how our health service works at the moment.

I understand that this means looking at the way we get help and care and how this has changed over the last two years.

For me, this means telling the researcher what I think and feel about how we get our care at hospital and at home.

Nothing I tell the researcher will be told to anyone else who knows it was me that said it, unless I say that is OK. I can stop being involved whenever I want and no one will mind.

Signed. . . . .

Name . . . .

Address . . . .

. . . .

. . . .

Witnessed by . . . .

Researcher . . . .

It must be pointed out, therefore, that you are conducting a research study and that individuals are never under any obligation to take part and have an absolute right to refuse. No inducement should be offered to take part, especially to vulnerable groups such as offenders or people in care, and it should never be implied that by co-operating with the research individuals will receive favourable consideration or treatment from staff. However, small gifts or monetary rewards for time taken can be offered to research subjects if this is appropriate and it is normal practice to pay expenses such as the reimbursement of travel costs to research subjects.

You should always remember that, just because you are carrying out a research study, even if you are a qualified health professional and have obtained ethical committee clearance as appropriate, you have no automatic right of access to research subjects or patients but need to remain polite and courteous in your requests for co-operation. This is important both for the sake of your own project and for the future of students and other researchers who may come after you. At the start of a study, the researcher should make it clear that subjects have a right to withdraw at any subsequent time. Subjects who fail to attend or who fail to respond to a questionnaire can be contacted again and invited to participate, but subjects must understand their right to refuse to continue with a research study at any stage.

Once data has been collected, the researcher has a duty not to disclose any information about identifiable individuals to any third parties. In the case of a student project which is supervised, your supervisors would not be regarded as third parties. In the project report, and any subsequent report or publication, the data should be presented in aggregate form, that is, as averages, totals and so on. If individual data is presented, this must not include information which could identify subjects. When the study is complete, any confidential information collected about individuals should be destroyed. If confidential information is collected, it is important that it is not left lying around in public places but kept securely in a locked place.

Assurances of confidentiality that you will be required to give at the outset of an investigation are normally binding on the researcher. Thus, as has been stated above, you should not disclose to a third party any information gained in confidence for research purposes. This confidentiality may be *absolute*, that is, no disclosure will ever occur, or it may be *conditional*, in which case conditions under which disclosure of information could occur must be explained to the participating subjects at the outset. Sometimes confidentiality may be breached accidentally, even though names and addresses may be withheld from reports. You need to be especially vigilant if you use a case study approach in your report.

Deception of subjects concerning the true purpose of the investigation should be avoided. In certain types of investigation this may be unavoidable. In these cases, the British Psychological Society guidelines state that:

> It may be impossible to study some psychological processes without withholding information about the true object of the study or deliberately misleading the participants. Before conducting such a study, the investigator has a special responsibility to (a) determine that alternative procedures avoiding concealment or deception are not available; (b) ensure that the participants are provided with sufficient information at the earliest stage; and (c) consult appropriately upon the way that the withholding of information or deliberate deception will be received.
>
> (Robson 1993:472)

Particular ethical difficulties are likely to arise for projects involving the use of psychiatric data about individuals or concerning offenders, children, older people with mental confusion or for experimental studies which could influence ongoing programmes of treatment. An ethics committee will need to be satisfied that there are real potential benefits of the research in these cases and why it is necessary to conduct the research with particular vulnerable groups. Otherwise, fairly harmless procedures such as interviewing could prove harmful or intrusive to some vulnerable individuals who may not be able easily to articulate their concerns. The question of informed consent needs to be carefully addressed in such studies, and every effort should be made to obtain the real consent of children and of adults with impairments in understanding or communication. Where this cannot be obtained, researchers should consult with someone who knows the person well, such as a member of the family.

If the above guidelines are adhered to and ethical committee permission obtained as necessary, there is less likelihood of any complaint being lodged concerning a research study. Even if ethical committee permission has been obtained, this does not absolve the researcher from personal responsibility should a complaint be made about the conduct of the research.

Research subjects or patients should be fully debriefed at the end of an investigation in order to pick up any unforeseen negative effects or misconceptions about the research. This is particularly important for laboratory or clinical investigations where people should not be left concerned about the outcomes. In addition, it is only courteous to supply a copy of the principal findings to managers or clinicians or others who have given permission and allowed the use of their facilities.

One of the principles upon which an ethics committee will make a decision is whether the study is deemed to be sound in its design and in the way it will be conducted. To conduct research involving human, or indeed animal, subjects other than by established investigative principles is unethical, since they may be exposed to potential harm for no good reason. These design principles are outlined in the next chapter of this handbook.

Action points

- Consider the ethical implications of what you intend to do.
- Ascertain whether local research ethics committee approval will be necessary.
- If you need ethics committee approval, find out when the appropriate committee meets and plan accordingly.

Chapter 3

Different questions, different designs ...

Like people, each piece of research is unique and requires an individual approach. A set of rules such as have to be followed, for example, for the emergency fire procedures in your workplace or for the assembly of a motor car are inappropriate if you wish to research the impact of handedness on dyslexia or the role of the advocate for people with learning difficulties. How you go about addressing the particular question, in the context in which you have encountered it, is up to you to approach in ways based on your experience, wisdom and creative vision. One of the exciting things about being a researcher is that boundaries only exist in order to be moved, and innovation and creative practice are positively encouraged when they lead to new insights. For these reasons, I would never encourage a 'cook book' approach to research or simplistic adherence to lists of Do's and Don't's which do not assist the process of genuine research. When I was a PhD student in a lab, our research group had a derogatory term to describe people (always from another lab, of course) who simply applied standard techniques to amass more and detailed information about a phenomenon: they were 'stamp collectors'.

There are recognised ways of carrying out research, and until you are thoroughly familiar with them, you will not be in a position to recognise and overcome their limitations. You should at least be familiar with the quantitative–qualitative distinction. To polarise the distinction, the former deals with numbers about phenomena which have been collected and the latter with the meaning of non-numerical data about phenomena. It is unfortunate in my opinion that this essentially methodological distinction has historically been associated with sometimes entirely different philosophical leanings. Thus it is not unusual for 'hard-nosed' statisticians to debunk the 'subjective' interpretations that the qualitative community work with, nor for qualitative advocates to decry the poverty of the data about phenomena which are dealt with by those who wish to quantify everything. Whilst science aims to understand by systematic enumeration and quantification of natural phenomena as a basis for deriving general rules, it may be appreciated that, in the field of health, this is by no means always possible – and many would argue that it is not even a desirable or feasible ultimate goal. Thus there is a great deal of truth in the saying that:

> Not everything that can be counted, counts
> And not everything that counts can be counted.

There are undoubtedly many aspects of the human experience which we know cannot be reduced to, or adequately described by, a set of numbers in a spreadsheet. Similarly, simply because something may be quantified does not in itself elevate its conceptual importance above qualitative data, however sophisticated the resulting statistical analysis might be. Indeed, many studies have shown 'statistically' significant findings which may have little or no practical or clinical importance. There is evidence of an increasing recognition of this amongst the research community and qualitative techniques have experienced an upsurge of interest in recent years. For example, health care providers who a few years ago would routinely conduct large scale quantitative surveys to assess consumer satisfaction or perceptions about services are increasingly turning to more qualitative approaches, such as focus group research, to address these issues.

At the risk of stereotyping, to physicists quantification is paramount whereas to the historian or the language scholar meaning and interpretation are all-important. In the field of health, there is adequate room for a plurality of approaches, including all recognised qualitative and quantitative methods, to the understanding of the human organism in its social and biological environment.

The range of research methods in health

Research studies in the field of health usually follow one of these ways of collecting data.

- laboratory experimental studies
- field clinical trials
- quasi-experimental studies
- cohort studies
- case–control studies
- surveys
- participant or non-participant observation studies
- focus group studies
- ethnographic field studies
- examination of records
- interview methods
- diary methods
- case studies.

It is not proposed to deal with each of these in detail here, but concepts in research design and practice appropriate to each may be consulted in many books listed in Chapter 18. In the above list, research studies which adopt a quantitative approach are generally placed in the first part whereas those adopting a qualitative method are placed in the second part of the list. You will see that surveys are deliberately placed towards the middle of the table and are widely employed across all the disciplines relating to health. The survey methodology is therefore examined first in more detail in the following section.

Surveys

Surveys are generally cross-sectional; that is, they occur at a single point in time and gain a snapshot of a dynamic situation, and they frequently employ a questionnaire. Questionnaires may use either closed questions, consisting of a limited and defined range of response options which generate quantitative data, or may use open-ended questions, which allow free text responses from participants, to generate data suitable for qualitative analysis. Questionnaire

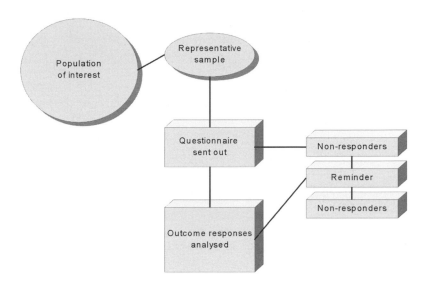

Figure 3.1   Design of a postal questionnaire survey.

design techniques are specifically covered in Chapter 5. A typical design of a postal question-naire survey is depicted in Figure 3.1.

The survey methodology is widely used by students conducting health-related projects. Generally speaking, a survey may be conducted relatively cheaply and easily compared to some other methods of data collection, at least on the scale encountered within a student project. First time researchers are generally more confident with the survey methodology than with many other types of study; we would have had to live a pretty hermit-like existence not to take part in many surveys during our lifetime. The survey generally collects structured information from individuals. Unlike the experimental methodology discussed below and in Chapter 6, the survey aims to be descriptive of a current situation and no interventions are carried out. Unlike experimental work, it is very difficult to determine cause and effect with a survey, although this is frequently attempted. Thus researchers have claimed on the basis of survey evidence, for example, that boys who watch Formula 1 racing are several times as likely to smoke cigarettes as boys who do not; this is a topical example at the time of writing. Whilst the claim may be true, the implication that cigarette advertising on racing cars influences boys to smoke does not follow. There may well be other factors, some of which the researchers may not even have assessed, such as personality differences between boys who are interested in motor racing and boys who are not, which may influence the relationship with smoking behaviour. Likewise, it would be erroneous to claim, if in a survey a link was discovered between ill-health and unemployment, that being out of work is detrimental to your health. Somebody else could claim that the evidence is equally consistent with the possibility that people who are not well have a harder time staying in employment and that the link is actually the other way round. Yet another argument might go something like this: there is no direct causal relationship at all between the two factors; unemployment and ill-health are really a reflection of two different aspects of a common factor which is low socio-economic status or deprivation. A third or common factor like this is called a 'confounding variable' by researchers. If your intention, therefore, is to try to link cause and effect in your study a survey

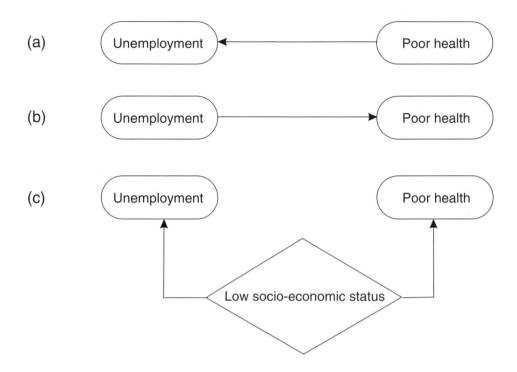

Figure 3.2   Explanations for a link between unemployment and ill-health.

methodology would not be the method to choose. The three alternative explanations put forward here are illustratrated in Figure 3.2.

Having recognised this, surveys have their place for the purposes of exploratory and descriptive research. They can generate a great deal of data on the views or attitudes of people about a topic and the relationship between these and various demographic characteristics of the responders, such as age, gender or employment status. Sometimes with such data, sophisticated statistical analyses are necessary to determine whether variables are being confounded and the usual cross-tabulation procedures which are frequently employed (see Chapter 8) may be inadequate. A major advantage of the questionnaire survey is that it enables data to be collected anonymously from individuals compared to, say, the experimental or interview approaches, and people may be willing to be more forthcoming about sensitive topics if they know they cannot be identified.

The response rate to a postal questionnaire may vary widely and is known to be influenced by a number of factors over which you have some control. I have conducted many surveys over the years and the following techniques are known to work. A single mailing to a group of respondents will bring a certain number of questionnaires back, whilst a reminder sent out perhaps two or three weeks after the initial mailing will bring in a further number. Sending a reminder is not possible in an anonymous survey, of course, as you have no way of determining who has replied and who has not. Sometimes a code number, disguised as a reference number perhaps on the return address, may help to identify respondents. An alternative is to send a reminder to the whole of the original sample with an instruction to ignore it if they have already sent back a questionnaire. A higher response rate is likely to be obtained if you write a polite and informative covering letter explaining the purpose of the research.

Even if you are sending out several hundred questionnaires, it is well worth the effort of personally signing each covering letter, since people are more likely to respond to this than to a letter sent out with a photocopied signature. It is well recognised that response rates are improved if you enclose a stamped self-addressed envelope, since returning the questionnaire does not involve respondents spending any money and because some people feel an obligation to use it if you have sent it. Even if an *sae* is sent along with a questionnaire, the name and address of the person to whom the questionnaire should be returned should be clearly stated on the instrument itself, since some envelopes will become separated from the questionnaires and if people have to go to the effort of looking for one they may not bother.

If you have access to an official organisation under whom the questionnaires can be sent out on headed paper, such as a Community Health Council or a voluntary sector organisation, this is likely to lead to a better response rate than questionnaires sent out under the name of an unknown individual. General guidance cannot be given on what is an 'acceptable' response rate in a survey, since this will depend upon a number of factors and whether procedures have been taken to compare the known characteristics of responders and non-responders. However, if less than half of the questionnaires sent out are eventually returned you might have serious doubts about the representative nature of the replies which have been received. That is, a response bias is always likely to be present in survey data so that people who return questionnaires may be more interested or have stronger feelings about the topic than those who do not. A response rate of sixty to seventy per cent from a survey is frequently found in published studies although, even at the upper end of this range, the influence of response bias needs to be seriously considered.

Selection bias may also be present in a survey if an inadequate sampling technique is employed. Selection bias implies that not everyone in the potential population has an equivalent chance of being included in the sample sent questionnaires, which can arise, for example, from a convenience sampling technique. Chapter 4 discusses these issues in some detail. In some projects it may be possible to survey the whole population of interest if this is a relatively small, well defined group such as consultants within a particular district or the pupils in a particular school. In most cases, however, a sample will need to be drawn from the population of interest and, if the responses from the sample are to be generalised to the whole population of interest, the sample will need to be representative. A representative sample may consist of a randomly selected percentage of the total population, in which case every individual in the population has an equal chance of being included in the sample. Sometimes a stratified random sampling method may be preferable. With this method, certain characteristics of the population will be accurately reflected in the sample which is not necessarily going to be the case in small samples taken at random. It may not be possible to obtain a representative sample for some kinds of survey research, for instance because there are no 'lists' of people from whom to draw a sample. Research with gay people or street drug users, for instance, has employed a 'snowball' sampling technique whereby a small number of initial contacts puts the researcher in touch with others and the sample accumulates that way. Issues concerned with sampling are dealt with in more detail in Chapter 4.

Experimental studies

The characteristic feature of an experimental study is that there is an active intervention by the researcher – in contrast to observational or descriptive studies such as surveys which have been considered above. The experimental method is appropriate for most laboratory studies where there is usually a random allocation of subjects to different conditions and ideally everything except the variable whose effects are being examined (the 'independent' variable) is held constant or controlled. Laboratory investigations are discussed more fully in Chapter 6. A randomised placebo-controlled clinical trial, such as a drug trial, is also an experimental procedure although normally conducted in the field. Those whose job it is to evaluate the evidence base of current medical practice, using techniques known as 'meta-analysis' (that is, weighing up and evaluating the findings from many different studies), have a 'pecking order' for the weighting which they apply to the evidence emerging from different types of research designs. At the top of the list, what is usually regarded as the 'gold standard' for clinical evidence is the placebo-controlled double blind randomised clinical trial (RCT). This is an experimental technique, as the levels of an independent variable – that is, the factor being altered such as the dosage of a drug – are manipulated in order to determine its effect on the outcome or dependent variable, such as the measured blood pressure. In an early trial, healthy volunteers would be employed and randomised to the active or placebo (dummy treatment) group. In a double blind trial, neither the researchers nor the subjects would be aware of which group they were in, to minimise unconscious, or conscious, bias and expectations concerning the outcome. It is usually regarded as 'hard' evidence of a cause-and-effect relationship if the drug emerges as better than the placebo under these circumstances.

It is recognised that volunteer bias is likely to exist in clinical trials; typically, poor socio-economic circumstances are related both to refusal to participate and to high risk, whereas volunteers may show lower risks. Random assignment in a clinical trial produces comparable groups although the drop-out rates may subsequently not be comparable, producing a potential bias. In recognition of this, data is sometimes analysed according to the way subjects were intended to be treated, whatever happened in practice. This is known as 'analysis by intention to treat', whereas analysing by treatment received is called 'on treatment analysis'. A typical design of a two group randomised controlled trial is depicted in Figure 3.3.

Although the experimental method, in the form of the RCT, is widely regarded as the 'gold standard' for evidence, this does not imply that other studies necessarily have inferior designs. The evidence from RCTs has been criticised on a variety of grounds.

- The research subjects are generally highly selected so that concurrent pathology is usually an exclusion criterion whereas, in practice in the 'real world', patients are not so homogeneous.
- Typically, the analysis of a trial involves the assessment of statistical significance of differences in the average responses between two (or more) groups. The variability of response that occurs *within each group* is often ignored or regarded as a statistical nuisance, but may be clinically important in practice.
- The dependent variables are usually a limited set of easily measurable outcomes but there may be other considerations surrounding the intervention. Quality of life assessments may also need to be conducted.

Thus, for example, clinicians have said to me that a new drug has not shown any difference in clinical trials from an alternative drug, but they know from clinical experience that the drug is

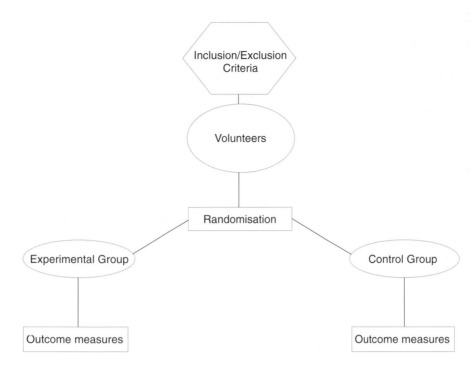

Figure 3.3   Design for a two-group randomised placebo-controlled clinical trial.

not indicated for certain types of patients. The argument has been articulated in a recent editorial in the *British Medical Journal* (BMJ 1999). In essence, the clinical trial gives information about whether something *can* work, under ideal and controlled circumstances. In practice, it may be a different matter whether is *does* work under usual circumstances and it is yet a further question whether it is worth it in terms of the patient gains against any costs, for example in resources and quality of life, of the intervention or treatment.

This particular argument is a specific instance of the more general consideration surrounding experimental studies involving people, and particularly laboratory-based studies that, in an attempt rigorously to control all extraneous variables, the researcher ends up losing 'ecological validity', that is, connection with the real-life situation. What is gained in control may be at the expense of the naturalness of the situation; this consideration needs to be seriously weighed in many psychological investigations where people often behave differently in the laboratory than they would in real life. In recognition of this, if your project involves, say, a controlled trial of the effects of a particular intervention – let us say a course of therapy sessions – my advice is to keep the trial as ecologically valid as possible consistent with the design of a randomised trial. Thus, for example, if a decision to stop the therapy would normally be made after certain clinical criteria have been achieved, use this as your end point for patients in the trial, so long as the criteria are agreed and specified in advance. The traditional experimental trial approach would be to continue the trial for a particular length of time with each patient given, say, a fixed number of sessions. Instead, by tailoring the design of a trial to the real-life situation, you are improving the chances of detecting effects and not reducing them by apparently losing elements of control.

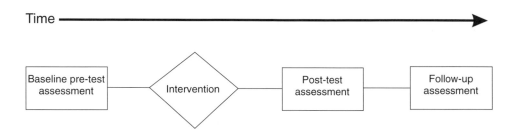

Figure 3.4   The design of a pre-test/post-test longitudinal intervention study without a control group but with a follow-up.

Quasi-experimental studies

Quasi-experimental studies involve examining the relationship between something that is being altered or changed (the independent variable) in the form of an intervention, and the eventual outcome of this (the dependent variable). However, unlike true experimental studies, certain aspects of control are absent, such as the allocation of subjects to groups, or a control group may be absent in some designs. Pre-test/post-test designs come into this group. For example, Figure 3.4 illustrates the design of a longitudinal action research study carried out in a community home for care of older people.

In the study illustrated in Figure 3.4, observational measurements were made of the levels of social interaction of the clients prior to the introduction of a new care programme (the pre-test or baseline measurements). Immediately following its introduction, the effects on the dependent variable (the amount of social interaction) were measured by the post-test assessment. To determine whether any measured differences were sustained, a third set of assessments was made three months later at follow-up. This is known as a repeated measures design using clients as their own controls. These designs suffer from a number of problems in practice.

- The dependent variable may change over time anyway. In the above example, the mix of clients and the staff can change over the period of the study which can affect social interaction irrespective of the intervention.
- Without a separate control group it is difficult to disentangle the effects of the intervention per se from the more general effects of taking part in a research study. This latter is known as the Hawthorne effect and may exert a considerable influence on the outcome.

To estimate the influence of the Hawthorne effect, it is normally always preferable to have a control group in intervention studies of this type. In the above example, the control could be another community home of similar size and matched as closely as possible on other relevant characteristics. The researchers would carry out all the baseline, post-test and follow-up observations in the same way as the experimental group but no intervention would occur, as is illustrated in Figure 3.5.

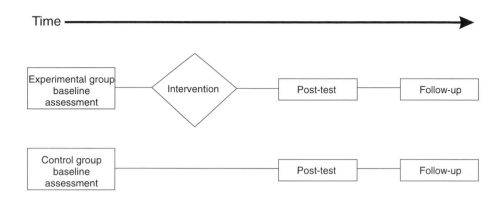

Figure 3.5   Design of a repeated measures intervention study with a control group.

Cohort studies

In the field of epidemiology, that is, the study of the distribution and determinants of disease generally at a population level, cohort studies are widely employed to help determine a link between morbidity (disease) or mortality (fatal outcomes) and aetiology (causes). Long term follow-up studies of the health outcomes of smoking or of eating a diet high in saturated fats are examples of cohort studies. In general, cohort studies follow a group of people sharing some characteristic (the 'cohort') over a period of time. They are therefore descriptive observational research designs, and there is no active intervention on the part of the researcher. Cohort studies are longitudinal studies and are normally prospective, that is, they start at one point in time and progress over a period of time, sometimes many years. A typical design of a cohort study is depicted in Figure 3.6.

Cohort studies tend to be expensive and they suffer from a number of recognised difficulties.

- There are problems of attrition of the original sample which gets smaller and smaller over time since people drop out, move away, die from unrelated conditions and so on, over the period of the study.
- The initial risk factor, or reason for the investigation, can alter as a result of changes in individuals' lifestyle, e.g. people may give up smoking.
- Cohort studies can require a long time to provide an answer to a question, so that a disease may only develop in the 'risk' group after many years of exposure and often a more immediate answer may be needed.

However, in terms of the 'hardness' of the evidence for cause and effect, cohort studies are regarded as coming close to placebo-controlled randomised experimental studies. They can provide an ethical alternative to a randomised controlled trial in order to determine cause and effect, for example whether there is a link between exposure to a hypothesised environmental hazard and a particular health outcome. Prospective cohort studies are usually the province of teams with available resources in the form of research grants and time available and are not usually a method suited to student project work, although a prospective study of this type could be carried out, given a carefully framed research question, within the limits of a programme of higher degree work.

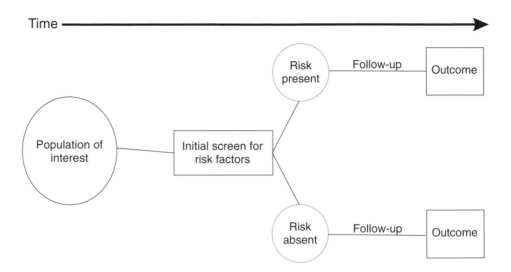

Figure 3.6   Design for an epidemiological cohort study.

Case–control studies

Case–control studies are a popular method of attempting to come to conclusions concerning the causes of health-related events. Cases of a particular problem or outcome are chosen and one or more controls without the outcome, but who may be matched in other respects such as age, gender and location, are chosen for each case. People in each group are then investigated as appropriate using interviews, analysis of medical treatment, life circumstances, examination of records and so forth. Case–control studies are very efficient at gaining such information about potential causes since the outcome has already happened, unlike the cohort method described in the previous section. However, they can suffer from a number of recognised biases in recall of information from individuals, perhaps relating to events occurring years before; also, medical records may be incomplete or inaccurate. This problem is particularly salient should there be reason to suspect that cases show differential recall compared to controls. Human memory can be highly selective and people tend mentally to 'link' events such as the development of impairment with particular circumstances, which may then be vividly recalled when no such causal connection existed.

A classic example of the case–control methodology was the thalidomide tragedy in the late 1950s. The medical records of a group of mothers (the cases) who had delivered a child with abnormal limbs were compared with normal controls, and it was found that the cases had much higher rates of having taken the drug thalidomide at certain critical stages of foetal development. A case–control study is therefore a retrospective design. A typical design of a case–control study is depicted in Figure 3.7.

One particular area of difficulty with case–control studies arises concerning the selection of the controls; the cases may be hospital patients with a particular diagnosis, but what should the controls be? They may be patients hospitalised with another diagnosis, in order to match certain characteristics associated with hospitalisation, or it may be more appropriate to use another control group, but often the decision is not straightforward. The case–control study

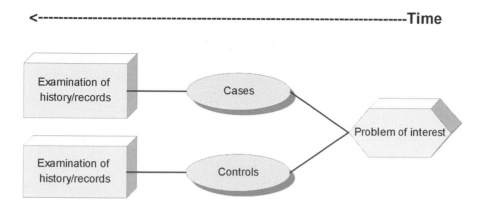

Figure 3.7   Design of a retrospective case–control study.

methodology is, however, within the bounds of practical methods available to the sole researcher on a limited budget and may be relatively simple and quick to conduct, depending upon availability and ease of access to the required records.

None of the foregoing arguments imply that the quantitative approach is paramount and should be the method of choice in health investigations. It is often not possible to experiment on people for a whole variety of ethical and practical reasons. Furthermore, and more substantively, the evidence from quantitative studies represents the overall statistical aggregation of data from a sample of people and the richness of individual description and variation is often lost. That is the province of the qualitative domain.

Observation and ethnography

Participant observation is a more qualitative technique than non-participant observation. The latter is frequently used by social psychologists and the aim is to have no effect on the behaviour being observed. As a result, many such studies take place in special rooms fitted with a one-way mirror. Non-participant observation frequently takes the form of recording data against predefined 'checklists' of behavioural patterns, sometimes using a variety of graphic symbols representing body positions. These structured observations may be augmented by still or video camera recording, audio recording or handwritten notes. If a group is being observed, there could be a systematic sequence of sampling which is applied to the observation, for example with each individual being observed for thirty seconds at a time. Some psychologists, however, object that behaviour is a complex interaction between individuals and cannot be reduced to the recording of units of behaviour on checklists. They argue that the meaning of the behaviour in the context in which it occurs should be the unit which is analysed. You need to decide, therefore, about the activity that is going to be recorded. This may include the content of verbal behaviour (what is said), the manner of verbal behaviour (how it is said), spatial behaviour (orientation and movement towards and away from others) and detailed aspects of non-verbal behaviour (frowns, direction of gaze, hand movements and so forth). You may be interested in recording the frequency with which particular events or units of behaviour occur, but what is often more informative is to record the timing and sequence of behaviour.

Issues surrounding the reliability of such data are concerned with the extent of agreement two or more observers would have in coding the same data (inter-rater agreement) and the consistency with which a single observer codes the same events or sequences on different occasions (intra-rater agreement). Both of these aspects of reliability may be checked fairly easily and are important aspects to be considered when employing the technique. The extent of agreement or concordance of two sets of such data can be checked by calculating the kappa statistic which has a value of one when agreement is perfect, whereas a value of zero indicates agreement no better than chance. A value above 0.8 is generally regarded as very good agreement, and kappa values below about 0.6 can be regarded as unsatisfactory consistency for observational studies.

It has been argued that more authentic observation of people within their network of relationships requires a less structured participant observational technique. Participant observation comes within the ambit of 'ethnographic' research methods. In one form of this, the role of the researcher is disguised and s/he becomes a member of the group studied. In other scenarios, the role of the researcher is recognised and members of the group accept the observer as a researcher. Clearly, it needs to be recognised that the presence of a participant observer may well change group behaviour. The participant observer does not usually take notes at the time, but may write up a detailed record book, say at the end of each day. The purpose of the ethnographic field study is to describe the characteristics and lifestyle of a group. This may be older people living in sheltered accommodation, drug self-injectors or New Age Travellers. The aim is to describe the characteristics of the group as faithfully as possible, using personal observation and ethnographic interview techniques. Unlike survey research, the principal aim may not be so much to examine influences and links between data but faithfully to record and describe group characteristics. The research method derives from anthropological roots and anthropologists like Malinowski and Margaret Mead published classic studies on far-flung societies in the Pacific and in Africa.

The ethnographic approach relies very much on the observations and interpretations of the researcher who does not use a structured recording technique, and as such is not an 'objective' scientific approach to data collection, using protocols and which can be repeated. In addition to observation, information is gained by speaking to members of the group using the ethnographic interview. This has been likened to the casual, friendly conversation with members of the group being studied. Different aspects of the interview methodology in the research context are dealt with in some detail in Chapter 9.

Focus groups

The focus group has in recent years gained great popularity as a qualitative method for investigating health and health care issues, and has a longer history as a market research technique. Focus group methodologies share some of the characteristics needed of the interview method, but whereas interviews are normally conducted with individuals, focus groups gather together a small group of people, no more than about eight to twelve, usually with some common interest, such as consumers of a service or as representatives of their peer group. A group facilitator aims to guide, to a greater or lesser extent, the agenda of the discussion. In respect of the process of moderating a focus group, Kreuger (1994) has written:

> Respect for participants may be one of the most important factors affecting the quality of focus group results. The moderator must truly believe that the participants have wisdom

no matter what their level of education, experience, or background. Indeed, they may have limited knowledge, hold opposing values to that of the researchers, or have fuzzy logic, but still the moderator listens attentively with sensitivity.

(Kreuger 1994:101)

Focus group methodologies have been used to augment quantitative data gained from a wider sample of the group of interest and in these circumstances can provide an opportunity for in-depth discussion around issues not possible through a questionnaire survey. Another way in which the focus group has proved of value has been to help identify starting points for research by revealing issues and concepts of which the researcher may not have been aware. They may be particularly valuable when there is a communication gap between different parties involved, such as professional groups (providers, doctors, technical groups and so on) and consumers or clients of services, and they can thereby assist the process of making services more 'consumer led'.

The principal advantages of the focus group technique can be summarised as economy of time and effort compared to individual interviews, and, more substantively, as providing an insight into the dynamics of attitudes and opinions in a group compared to more rigid questionnaire studies. These dynamics are a key element of the success, or otherwise, of a focus group session. Thus focus group research needs to guard against the potential difficulty that its results are very much the product of the mix of individuals present. A potential bias could be introduced into the conclusions should there be one or two particularly vocal individuals who may articulate some arguments. The lack of discussion or objection from other individuals does not necessarily imply their assent although this could be inferred. It is a role of the group facilitator not to let arguments automatically hold sway through their power of articulation by dominant individuals. If a consensus is achieved in a group this may reflect the group dynamics but, unlike the interview situation, is unlikely to reflect the subtleties of individual range of opinion on an issue. The danger of drawing wrong conclusions may be reduced if more than one focus group is held, with different participants, and this is a recommended method of increasing the reliability of focus group research.

Although focus group members are not intended to be a 'representative' sample in the same way that a survey methodology would aim at, there are criteria which apply to the selection of focus groups attendees. Thus the characteristics of the people in the group need to be identified in order to avoid an obvious selection bias. Selection bias can emerge by selecting group members through personal contacts, because individuals have expressed some particular concern or feel strongly about a topic, or because they have some strong vested interest in the topic area under discussion. The aim is usually to obtain a balanced selection of members who are likely to represent different views.

The degree to which focus group findings may be generalised is rather less than, say, for a survey involving a random sampling technique (see Chapter 4). It has been argued, however, that theoretical generalisation may be possible. Here, theoretical insights into a situation may be gleaned through the technique which may be projected to other contexts or situations. Thus it may be possible to recognise conceptual parallels between situations rather than basing generalisation upon considerations of quantitative extrapolation. That is, you may not be so sure after a focus group study that, say, 25 per cent of the participants agree with a certain view compared to a survey methodology, but the process and dynamics of attitude formation within a defined set of contexts on the issue may be much clearer and be capable of wider application beyond the individuals in the group.

Other qualitative methods

Diaries, as records of activities, are another qualitative data source in health research. Subjects themselves may be asked to keep such a log of thoughts or feelings, for example, at regular intervals or associated with activities of interest to the study. Diaries may, however, be onerous and distracting for the participants, who can also introduce their own biases into a study. People may be unwilling to record activities which may be regarded as socially unacceptable, for instance; also, the process of keeping a diary will influence their actions. A diary may be kept over a negotiated time period, perhaps a week or month. A major problem is deciding how to analyse the wealth of often detailed information produced from diaries. One method which is sometimes adopted is to request that the participants produce information in set ways so that categories can be generated and subsequently analysed from the resulting data.

The analysis of documents draws upon research techniques which historians frequently use. Thus it may be necessary to verify the authenticity and establish the validity of documentary sources before admitting them as evidence. Questions surrounding the purpose of the document, the completeness of the documentation as well as its content may need to be addressed. The context in which the document was produced may be critical to its interpretation; if it consists of the minutes of primary health care team meetings, for example, are they an accurate reflection of the discussions at the meetings or have they been 'massaged' for publication? Judith Bell writes of such documents:

> If you detect bias, that does not necessarily mean that the document should be dismissed as worthless. Inferences can still be drawn from the 'unwitting' testimony, even if the 'witting' evidence is thought to be unsound. A prejudiced account of curriculum development for example could provide valuable insights into the political processes involved in innovation. The biased document will certainly need to be analysed cautiously and compared with evidence from other sources, but it can still be valuable.
>
> (Bell 1993:72)

Writing individual case studies is another recognised type of research activity in the field of health. Thus the leading medical journals such as the *Lancet* and the *British Medical Journal* frequently publish the history, diagnostic signs and treatment of unusual cases or manifestations of some disease, and they can be clinically valuable. The case study approach is perhaps the least generalisable of the methods used by researchers; the aim is generally not to say a lot about a group but to describe the experiences of individuals. A series of case studies, however, may be collected, such as on the experiences of older people on discharge from hospital, and if patterns emerge these findings may be generalisable. The case study may use observation, interview, clinical assessment, diaries or a range of other techniques as appropriate.

Choosing a methodology

There may be a number of alternative approaches which you could adopt for a study. The choice of method or combination of methods adopted is likely to depend a great deal on the particular question being addressed. For example, a psychological investigation aimed at examining the extent to which reaction times may be influenced by cognitive processing clearly points to a controlled experimental methodology. A comparison of the lifestyles of young people in different parts of the UK points to a comparative survey, although you might consider supplementing the questionnaire data with a focus group approach. An examination and exploration of the experiences of psychiatric patients on discharge from hospital could point to a qualitative interview approach, and so on. The decision on methodology will also be influenced by factors such as whether you have a specific hypothesis to investigate, whether you wish to extend or question the findings of another study and the resources and expertise available, as well as the personal preferences of the researcher. Whatever method of data collection is adopted, a sample of research subjects will be required. The next chapter therefore discusses in some detail considerations in choosing a sample.

Action points

- Consider alternative ways of addressing the research question of interest and decide on one or more methods, depending upon the purposes of the investigation.
- Recognise the strengths and weaknesses of each of the research methods and consider how the weaknesses might affect your particular study.

Chapter 4

Choosing a sample

Whatever method of approach is adopted in a research study, consideration will need to be given to choosing an appropriate sample. For some studies, the entire population of interest may be included, if the population is a narrowly defined group, such as nurses working within a local hospital. Normally, however, a proportion of the entire population of interest is selected and this involves choosing a sample. Sometimes a list of the names and addresses of the population of interest is available, such as all patients registered with a local general practice. The electoral register, which is a publicly available document, provides another source of potential names and addresses for the adult general population. Very often, of course, such ready made lists of the potential population of interest, such as self-injecting drug users, gay people or past users of mental health services, are simply not available.

Defining the population of interest, therefore, will help establish the type of sampling technique which may be used. Another consideration is the nature of the study, so that a survey may require a different sampling technique from an experimental study or a qualitative study. There are fundamentally two different sorts of sampling procedures, although many variations exist within each broad grouping. These have been called probability samples and non-probability samples.

Probability samples

A probability sample aims to be representative of the population of interest; a straightforward random sample involves, statistically speaking, putting the names of every member of the population into a hat and randomly drawing a fixed proportion such as 5 or 10 per cent. The characteristic of this type of random sample is that each individual in the population has an equal chance of being included. In practice, due to the inaccuracies of ready made lists, it is often extremely difficult to draw a random sample of a population. If the population is therefore the general adult population in a certain area, neither the electoral register nor lists of those registered with local general practitioners will provide a random sample; homeless and itinerant groups, for example, will be greatly under-represented in such lists and this may be important for many health-related studies.

Other types of probability samples include stratified samples, systematic samples and cluster samples. A true random sample will not guarantee that the proportions of sub-groups in the sample will be the same as that existing in the entire population. For example, if the proportion of males and females in the population of interest is, say, 11:10, a 10 per cent random sample may end up with a different distribution, purely by chance say, 12 of one gender and 9 of the other. That is the 'luck of the draw' with a random sample; having said this, the probability of getting a very different distribution from that existing in the population is statistically small. However, where it may be important to guarantee a proportionate representation of sub-groups a stratified random sampling procedure may be undertaken. The population is first divided or stratified into each group and the same random proportion is then drawn from each group. A disproportionate stratified random sampling technique is a variation on this procedure. For example, if it was desired to survey the views of the staff of a local Trust stratified by staff occupational grouping, a 10 per cent stratified random sample may produce a sample containing many nurses, managers and junior doctors but only a very small number of consultants, and in order to get a broader range of consultants' views, 20 per cent of the consultants may be selected randomly.

A systematic sample is produced by choosing individuals from a predefined list at fixed intervals. Thus, every fifth person on a list may be selected or every tenth house in a locality may be visited. This method is sometimes used because it is often easier to arrange in practice and may be based upon the assumption that it will produce a sample which is as representative as a true random sample. However, this may not be the case and it is normally preferable to use a method where every individual has an equal chance of being included.

Another proportionate sampling technique is the cluster sample. This involves partitioning the population of interest into a number of clusters, each containing individuals with characteristics of interest to the study within a particular district, a number of general practitioners could be selected randomly and then, from each of these GP lists, all patients will be selected to take part in the study. This differs from a true random sample in that patients at all practices in the district will not have an equal chance of inclusion and so, strictly speaking, the results may only be generalised to the patients at the practices actually selected. A variation on the cluster sampling technique involves a multi-stage sampling so that, in the above example, from the lists of patients at the doctors chosen, a random sample of patients will be chosen. It is potentially possible to combine some of these proportionate sampling methods so that a stratified multi-stage sample could be selected.

Table AIII.1 in Appendix III may be used to draw a sample from a predefined list or else randomly to allocate subjects to groups in an experimental study. In the table, each number appears equally often and there is no ordering or sequencing in the digits. The way to use a table of random numbers is to take an arbitrary starting point and then work upwards, downwards or across in either direction. If the need is to allocate, say, to two groups in an experiment, this could be achieved in a number of different ways using the table. For example, even digits could represent group 1 and odd digits group 2. If the need is to allocate to three groups, numbers up to 0.3333 could be used for group 1, between this value and 0.6666 for group 2 and the remainder up to 0.9999 for group 3.

As has been pointed out above, drawing a sample through a process of pure randomisation will not necessarily result in the population characteristics being accurately reflected in the sample, and this is especially true when small samples are drawn. Thus, if there were, say, 100 males and 100 females in the population of interest and the need was to draw a 10 per cent sample, you could do this by allocating each person a number from 1 to 200 and randomly drawing 20 numbers within this range with the aid of Table AIII.1. If you wished to draw numbers within the range up to 200, you could use the table in the following way. Group the numbers into groups containing three digits, perhaps working downwards in the table. If the three digits are within the range up to 0.200, accept this number. If the digits make a number above 0.200, reject the number and move down to the next group of three digits. Do not forget to include leading zeros in your grouping of the numbers.

If it is necessary accurately to reflect some population characteristics, a different process is required. A sample can first be stratified, or grouped, into characteristics and then a separate random sample is drawn from each group. In the above example, 10 males and 10 females would each be randomly drawn. Further levels of stratification can occur so that stratification for both gender and age groups may be desirable, although it is not advisable to have more than one or two levels of stratification in a small study, since there may only be small numbers of subjects available at each stratum.

Another way of drawing a random sample may be more appropriate depending upon the nature of the task. If you had access to 2,000 manual patient records filed by surname from a GP practice and wished to draw a 5 per cent random sample (100 patients), one way this could be achieved would be to choose random numbers ranging from 0 to 40 in the way that I have described. These will be uniformly distributed over this range. By choosing cards according to this random sequence, that is, skipping between 0 and up to 40 records at a time, you should end up with one twentieth (5 per cent) of the cards selected. This will generate a random selection, whereas choosing every twentieth card will produce a systematic sample. In practice, the difference could be important. For example, runs of names vary in frequency so that there may be a lot of Jones' or Llewellyn's in a Welsh practice, some of whom would be certain to be chosen by the systematic method, whereas uncommon names, perhaps foreign names, would not. With a random sample, everybody has an equal probability of being included.

Non-probability samples

Non-probability samples generate samples where it is not possible to calculate the probability whereby any individual will be included in the sample. They are commonly used, for example, to select samples for pilot studies or where a particular purpose is in mind in some qualitative research. Unlike probability samples, generalisation to a population of interest is not clearly indicated. One method is the convenience sample. This is produced, for example, where individuals are stopped on the street and asked questions in a survey. Another type of convenience sample is generated where a researcher contacts colleagues who may be working in the area of interest. A further example of a convenience sample is generated where a researcher puts a notice on boards seeking volunteers to take part in an study. It needs to be recognised that convenience samples may produce seriously biased data. In a street survey involving daytime interviewing, for example, people in full time employment are going to be under-represented, the housebound and institutionalised will not be represented, and so forth. Convenience sampling may, however, be acceptable if the aim is to do an initial exploratory study to gain an understanding of the range of opinion on an issue or to pilot methods.

Quota sampling is a more systematic approach to non-probability sampling than convenience sampling. It appears initially akin to the stratified sampling technique that has been discussed but, unlike that method, does not involve any random selection. The purpose of this method is to ensure representation of different groups in the population of interest. In a study concerned with examining the attitudes of hospital doctors, for example, 30 subjects may be selected to represent each of the groups of house officer, senior house officer and specialist registrar, making a total sample size of 90. Subjects are then chosen on a non-random basis, perhaps on a convenience basis, until the quota for each group has been allocated. Like the convenience sample, quota samples are subject to bias in the way the sample is selected.

The snowball sampling technique has been employed where it may be difficult or impossible to gain a sample by any other means. This principle relies on a few initial contacts each putting the researcher in touch with further subjects so that the sample accumulates over time in an unpredictable way. It has been used extensively to research sensitive issues such as sexual health, primarily in the context of a qualitative interview methodology.

Another type of sampling used in some qualitative approaches is the purposive sample. Here, a purpose is in mind in the selection of subjects for recruitment to the study. The sample is deliberately chosen, therefore, on the basis that the data which will be provided will be of central interest to the study. A grounded theory approach may start off with a small initial sample and then, on the basis of the initial results, further subjects will be chosen to augment and further examine various issues or theories which are emerging. This type of research aims to address the external validity – that is, the generalisability to a wider group – of the conclusions and interpretations through different means other than the selection of random samples and is a very different approach from the statistical approach. In addition to the sampling methods discussed above, other types of samples have been used for particular purposes. Thus individuals have been selected because they may have certain characteristics in common or not in common (homogeneous or heterogeneous samples) or because of geographical or temporal characteristics which may be of interest to the study.

Sample sizes

A question frequently asked is, 'What is the best, or alternatively the minimum, sample size to use?' In a qualitative project, adopting perhaps a grounded theory approach (see Chapter 10) to developing a theoretical perspective, the analysis may be based on as few as half a dozen interview transcripts, which may be examined and re-examined at great length. A prevalence study in the community may require a random sample of 500 or more if the prevalence of the condition is say 5 per cent (this will generate about 25 cases), and an even larger sample will be required if it is a rare condition. Many lifestyle surveys which are carried out have involved many thousands of respondents. The ideal sample size for a piece of research depends upon a number of factors: the purpose of the study, the size of differences to be expected between groups, the power of statistical tests used, the research design, the likely sampling error to be encountered and so on. A pilot study will help establish some of these factors.

As a general rule, it will require fairly marked differences to be present between groups for statistical tests to be useful with very small sample sizes. Sometimes sample sizes are chosen because they represent what appears to be a reasonable number, or because they represent the maximum number of cases that can reasonably be processed given the time and resources available. It should be appreciated, however, that many studies are inconclusive because of insufficient sample size. So a trend in the data might have become statistically significant if a larger sample had been used and the same differences had been measured. On the other hand, a sample which is too large will be a waste of resources and may be unethical if participants are potentially being exposed to some harm. There are recognised techniques for calculating an ideal sample size for a particular study which depend on estimates of the likely size of the effects being measured and the variability of the data.

Generally, in experimental and survey research, the more variable the data from individuals, the larger the sample size will need to be reliably to detect the differences between groups. Generally, the larger the effects being determined the smaller the sample size that may be used, given a certain degree of variability. For particular analyses there may need to be a minimum number of observations and this may help determine a minimum sample size in survey work. These factors may be estimated from initial pilot studies. Altman (1991) discusses the

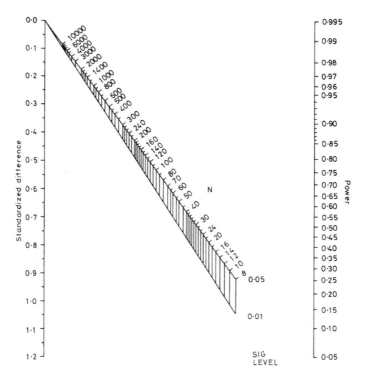

Figure 4.1   Nomogram for calculation of sample size (reproduced with permission from Altman 1991).

use of a nomogram for the purpose of calculating an ideal sample size. In principle, the method relies on calculating an ideal sample size based on the precision desired in an estimate of a population mean, the degree of confidence with which we wish to make the estimate and the amount of variability in the data. The nomogram is reproduced here in 4.1.

Assuming a study was being conducted with two groups involving a continuous dependent variable, the nomogram would be used in the following way. The standardised difference is calculated based upon the size of the difference expected or of interest between the two groups, divided by the standard deviation. For example, initial pilot work has indicated that increases in aerobic capacity of around 4 measured units compared to a control group were associated with an exercise regime and that the standard deviation (see Chapter 7) in the sample was around 5 measured units. The standardised difference in this case is therefore 4/5 = 0.8. The sample size required to detect a difference of this size with that variability depends first on the power of detecting the difference and second on the level of statistical significance (see Chapter 7) we wish to set. Normally, these calculations are made setting a power ranging from 80 to 95 per cent or so. Let us take 90 per cent as our required power level. Join up the value of the standardised difference, i.e. 0.8, with the 90 per cent power level using a straight edge such as a sheet of paper, and, at the 5 per cent (0.05) level of significance, the required total sample size (*n*) from the nomogram is about 64 subjects, or about 32 in each of the experimental and control groups. To detect this difference at the 1 per cent (0.01) significance level at the same power, the nomogram indicates that about 45 subjects would be required in each group.

Survey research generally aims to have high external validity or generalisability of the results; that is, the results are applicable beyond the individuals surveyed. Survey researchers, therefore, pay particular attention to their method of sampling and aim to get close to random samples of the population of interest. Experimental studies, as indicated in Chapter 6, tend to be more concerned with internal validity – that is, the results are true for the group studied – and cause and effect relationships, and frequently rely on volunteers for subjects, although great efforts may then be made randomly to allocate to experimental conditions. In contrast to both of these approaches, qualitative research frequently does not employ random selection or allocation and the aim may be adequately to describe and interpret the experiences of individuals in a case study approach, again with the emphasis on internal validity. Whatever sampling method you adopt will, however, need to be justified in relation to the aims and objectives of the study.

Action points

- Choose a recognised sampling method for your study based upon the type of research and the purpose of the study, as well as practical considerations such as the accessibility of potential research subjects.
- Decide on the appropriate number of research subjects needed for your study based on estimates from pilot work.

Chapter 5

There are more questions than answers ...

The need to develop a questionnaire is so often encountered in project work that it is worth devoting some special consideration to this widely used but frequently misunderstood procedure. It is common practice for students to devise their own questionnaires for survey research. In many cases, for example questionnaires which are designed to measure some aspect of health status, it would be better to employ a standard instrument to measure this: see the McDowell and Newell (1996) and Bowling (1997) volumes listed in Chapter 18. In the event that no suitable questionnaire is available, psychologists in particular have devised sets of procedures and principles for the construction of test instruments.

Do not be tempted to include items of casual or marginal interest to the nature of the study on the assumption that 'it might be useful'. If respondents cannot appreciate a focus to a questionnaire they are likely to be irritated, and in any case it is good practice to aim for the minimum length in a questionnaire which will fulfil the purpose of the investigation. Do not ask questions which are likely to be difficult to answer. This advice might appear obvious, but in many student questionnaires I have seen questions along the lines of 'Do you know what is the proportion of people over 65 affected by depression in the UK?', with the options ranging from something like 1 to 90 per cent. If you think about it, the overwhelming majority of people are only going to be able to hazard a guess at an answer. It is not surprising, therefore, that the findings of studies including such questions usually reveal a great deal of 'ignorance' on the part of the public, or whatever other group is being studied. But it is not only technical questions of which respondents can fall foul. An apparently simple question like 'How many times have you visited your GP in the last year?' would have many people stumped.

Only include questions which are likely to be answered honestly and accurately. Asking about alcohol consumption, for example, is a well known area where respondents may be economical with the truth. However, there are many other topics where respondents, even in anonymous questionnaires, may be inclined to give socially acceptable or expected answers rather say than how they really feel.

It is my experience that it is best to avoid the use of items like 'Rank the following list of symptoms in order of importance ...'. Many individuals, including highly educated people, find this a difficult and confusing task and instead of producing the desired pattern, e.g. 3, 4, 6, 1, 5, 2 for the six items will write something like 1, 1, 2, 3, 3, 3; that is, they will feel unable to discriminate between some items and give them equal ranking. Alternatively, they may leave out a ranking for some items altogether. This is likely to make the analysis of the ensuing data less than straightforward.

The ordering of questions and the layout of items in a questionnaire are matters that require careful thought. Groups of questions should be logically arranged around themes and topics with one question leading to another. There should be no repetition of essentially the same items, except in the special case where these are deliberately included in order to help assess reliability, that is, the internal consistency of an instrument. It is good practice to make the layout of the questionnaire as straightforward and simple as possible. Sometimes it may be necessary to include 'cut-off' questions such as 'Have you visited an outpatient department in the last 6 months?' Then if the answer is 'No', this may lead to the instruction 'Please go on to Section 2 of this questionnaire'. However, any 'routeing' around the questionnaire of this sort should be kept to the absolute minimum in self-completed instruments, and there should be no jumping backwards as well as forwards. The simple reason is that a proportion of the respondents will fall foul of the instructions; they will end up answering questions inappropriately or, worse, fail to answer questions you would wish them to.

Where in a questionnaire you put the demographic questions, that is, the general questions about gender, age, employment status and so on, is also important. Some authorities argue that they naturally come first, and that at least this important information is 'in the bag' even if other sections are not answered completely. However, do not dismiss the idea of putting them last, especially if other 'general' questions are to be included in that section, such as information about annual income which may have a better chance of being answered after the respondent's confidence has been gained and they can see a purpose to the questions. In the demographic section, it is common practice to ask for information about marital status and we have all seen questionnaires *ad nauseam* which include this item. If you think about it, it is rare indeed for a study to be influenced by whether or not a respondent is divorced, widowed, separated, single etc., and in any case this only provides information concerning the legal marital status of respondents. What the health researcher is often interested in is whether an individual has social or family support, but in the twenty-first century this information will certainly not be obtained by asking whether they are legally married or single. So leave it out.

Even if a questionnaire consists entirely of closed questions, it is always very good practice to include a space for comments, usually near the end, to give people a chance to express themselves verbally about an issue. Even if you do not intend to do any sophisticated qualitative analysis of the comments, most people will appreciate being invited to express their opinions in this way. Many student questionnaires in the health field deal with sensitive or 'difficult' topics. These items need to be carefully introduced and not just 'spring up' out of context. The researcher in these areas, for example in sexual health or mental health, needs especially to gain the confidence of the respondents that this is a serious and worthwhile study.

Most questionnaire instruments use closed response questions, since the data they generate can easily be coded and entered onto the computer and become subject to statistical analysis. On the other hand, it has, of course, been argued that open-ended questions, where there are no options but a space is provided for respondents to provide an answer in their own words, provide richer information and do not frustrate respondents by constraining the choices. As a general rule, I would suggest that it is advisable to stick with closed response type questions but leave the option of including some open-ended responses where this is appropriate, notably to encourage respondents to amplify their responses or explain reasons for a choice. The analysis of the data from some open-ended questionnaires may involve little more than attempting to classify the resulting textual responses into a set of categories and counting up the number of responses falling within each category. If this is what is envisaged, it is a tedious and unreliable task and the task could be essentially obviated through pilot studies which would help establish the necessary categories in the first place for a closed questionnaire.

Response formats can be varied as appropriate, for example as shown on page 36.

Binary: Yes ___

                        No _✓_

Do remember to include in addition an 'Unsure' or 'Don't know' option where this may be needed.

List of Categories: Why did you register with your present GP?

                        Only practice in the area ___

                        The nearest practice _✓_

                        Personal recommendation ___

                        The facilities available ___

                        Some other reason (*please state what below*)

Ordinal Scale: My age group is:

                        Under 16 years ___

                        16–25 years ___

                        26–35 years _✓_

                        36–45 years ___

                        46–55 years ___

                        56–65 years ___

                        Over 65 years ___

Free Response: I am ___ years old.

Analogue Rating Scale: How much pain did you experience immediately after the operation?

                        _____|_____

                        None   As much as imaginable

Five Point Likert Scale: Five point scale of this form:

                 Strongly agree Agree Undecided Disagree Strongly disagree
                 [ ]   [✓]   [ ]   [ ]   [ ]

Semantic Differentials: Bipolar adjectives of this form:

                        How are you feeling now?

                        excited _ _ _ ✓ _ _ _ bored

                        happy _ _ _ ✓ _ _ _ sad

                        calm _ _ ✓ _ _ _ _ anxious

There do exist a number of other possible ways of organising response formats for question-naire items which psychologists and social researchers have devised, but the above are the more commonly encountered ones. A few words are necessary concerning the choice from these various options. You should not mix too many types of scale in the same questionnaire, but if you do mix scales, keep all items using, for example, Likert scales together in one sec-tion. Both the Likert and the semantic differential scales illustrated above have as a feature a middle or 'undecided' point, but sometimes it is desirable to force respondents to choose one way or another; these are known as 'forced choice' scales and might consist of two positive and two negative scale points (4 point instead of a 5 point scale). If you do this, bear in mind that some respondents may simply omit answering the item altogether.

The main advantage of the visual analogue rating scale is that it generates a different type of data, that is, measurements on a ratio scale, usually on a scale of 0–100 mm measured with a ruler from the zero point. An advantage is, therefore, that you can employ more sophisticated statistical analyses. A further advantage is that, in principle, this type of scale should be the most sensitive to the detection of small degrees of change in respondents' responses over time when measured on separate occasions. It needs to be said, however, that some authorities do not like these scales for several reasons. One objection which a statistician voiced to me is that respondents are being asked to make precise judgements about something which may be quite subjective and that the data can therefore appear to have a spurious precision which is not really there. Another difficulty is that respondents are assumed to be using the scale in a con-sistent linear way (which is what treating the data as ratio scale measurements assumes) but they may not be doing this, and may even interpret the same scale in different ways on differ-ent occasions. Data obtained using these scales is also very often, in my experience, skewed in nature – that is, tends to be bunched up at one end – and may not therefore be analysed using sophisticated statistics anyway, so it may have been better to have used a fixed point scale, such as a 5 point scale, in the first place.

In the construction of attitude scale statements, or indeed any questionnaire items, you should avoid introducing complexity, such as long, convoluted statements with which respon-dents are being asked to agree or disagree. Technical terms, double negatives and ambiguity are also to be avoided. There is a recognised procedure for the development of attitude scale items in order to construct a Likert scale instrument. The first stage is to generate an equal number of favourable and unfavourable statements about the phenomena, bearing in mind the points mentioned above, and to refine these through a process of pre-piloting. A pilot study is then carried out where data is collected from a sample using the scale points illustrated above. An item analysis test should then be conducted in order to determine the most discriminating items. This should result in rejection of low discrimination items and the final version is pro-duced with a balance of favourable and unfavourable items arranged in a random or alternat-ing order. Items are considered good in a questionnaire if they discriminate well between respondents. This can be assessed by calculating correlations, that is, statistical associations, obtained from the pilot study, between each person's score on each item and their score on the test as a whole; high correlations provide discriminating items. This procedure is certainly not beyond the remit of student project work.

Other general principles which apply to the wording of questionnaire items include the need to avoid leading questions, that is, questions which it is difficult to avoid agreeing or dis-agreeing with, and the need to avoid biased, value loaded or emotive terms. Questionnaires and attitudinal scales can certainly be constructed where the outcome may be manipulated by the researcher in almost any desired direction by means of the selection and particular wording of items. The value of these instruments, of course, as tools of systematic investigation is virtually worthless. Another very common mistake is to ask essentially two questions rolled into one, or alternatively to make two separate points in the same attitudinal statement, e.g. 'The doctors at this surgery are excellent and never make mistakes.' It is perfectly possible for some respondents to wish to agree with the first part of the statement but to feel inclined to disagree with the second, resulting in confusion over how they should respond.

Any worthwhile instrument should be subject to checks of its reliability and validity. There are a number of recognised ways of checking reliability and validity, although it is regrettable that these aspects are only rarely properly investigated in student project work. An instrument which consists of a number of related items or questions can be split into two, providing two half instruments. This can be done after the data has been collected, and is a quick and easy way to check internal reliability; the extent of agreement of the two halves can be calculated and this is known as split half reliability. Test–retest reliability involves calculating the extent to which scores obtained on two different occasions with the same group of people are correlated. This is much more difficult to assess than internal reliability since there may be other factors which will influence people's scores the second time around.

There are many approaches to checking validity of an instrument. Many student questionnaires rely on face validity, that is, the questionnaire appears to look as if it is asking questions about the topic you are interested in, but this is a subjective measure providing no empirical evidence of validity. To go a stage further is very often not difficult, however, and this could involve a more comprehensive examination of content validity, that is, ensuring that the instrument contains questions on each dimension or factor important to the study. This may be established through procedures including a literature review and the Delphi technique. This latter involves recruiting an informed panel, perhaps of professional colleagues, who will sit down and examine an instrument. Criterion validity may be assessed if there exists another standard by which to compare the findings of your questionnaire, but very often there is not.

Construct validity, however, can be used to establish validity where no other measure exists. For example, the construct validity of a general practice patient satisfaction questionnaire was established by putting forward the construct that dissatisfied patients will be more likely than satisfied patients to change their doctors, without changing their address. When the performance of the instrument was compared from two groups of patients, those who had changed doctors and those who had not, the construct was borne out. This was taken as evidence that the questionnaire was able to detect dissatisfaction and so achieved high construct validity. It is not beyond the scope of a student project to check construct validity of a self-devised questionnaire in this way, and if these procedures are undertaken they should considerably strengthen the conclusions you may be able to come to concerning the study.

Although questionnaires are very commonly employed in research, many biological and psychological projects in particular rely on other ways of collecting data, especially experimental methods. These are introduced in the next chapter.

A note on psychometrics

Psychometrics (literally 'measuring the mind') gained great credence as an approach to developing assessment instruments by psychologists in the early decades of the twentieth century. A principal technique employed in the development of these instruments was factor analysis. This technique has been widely employed to determine a single underlying hypothetical construct, or factor, which is identified as underpinning a wide range of test performance. For example, this factor for general intelligence was named 'g'. Similarly, the investigation of personality questionnaires identified a number of factors – such as extroversion and neuroticism – which could account for particular patterns of responding. The extent to which individual items on a test instrument are associated – or 'load' on the factors – can be calculated, and this statistical procedure can therefore help to devise instruments with greater discriminative power for the factors investigated.

The extent to which questionnaire items are tapping into the same construct is therefore one use of factor analysis. A corollary is that 'redundant' items can be removed and factor analysis can thereby help generate instruments with a minimum number of variables. A factor analysis can be conducted on a set of questionnaire item responses by initially calculating a matrix of correlations between all the variables. If significant correlations exist – and they usually do – a factor analysis may then be conducted. If this stage is contemplated, a large data set is recommended; it would be misleading to conduct the analysis on 30 or 40 respondents. As a general rule of thumb, there should be considerably more cases than there are variables and a minimum of 100 cases has been proposed for a factor analysis. A factor analysis will enable the amount of variability explained by each factor to be determined. The first few factors are regarded as the most important; that is, they will explain a greater proportion of the variability than a single variable alone. It is common practice to go on and rotate the factors which have been identified to maximise the associations, or loadings, of some of the items in the instrument. There are various methods of rotation which can keep the factors independent of each other or related to each other.

It needs to be stressed that factor analysis is a technique capable of abuse; although the data resulting from such an analysis appears 'hard', the technique is based upon many subjective assumptions. Thus the interpretation or meaning of an identified factor is a subjective process which depends on knowledge of the items loading most highly upon it, and also on theoretical orientation. There is no unique solution from a process of factor analysis, and fundamentally, the technique can be used statistically to 'confirm' the existence of constructs which are just that – hypothesised aspects of the operation of mind which are merely one way of interpreting human responses. The process underlies a reductionist and mechanistic approach to the explanation of human performance and behaviour, and the interpretation of factor analytic studies should always bear this in mind.

Action points

- Use standard instruments with known validity and reliability if possible for your study, and only supplement these with a self-devised instrument where necessary.
- Give careful thought to the layout, appearance and design of your questionnaire.
- Decide on the form of the fixed choice questions, taking into account the considerations outlined in this section.
- Pilot any self-devised instrument carefully and use the results to inform an improvement.
- Check the reliability and validity of your questionnaire.

Chapter 6

Working in the lab

Experimental studies, at least as much as observational ones, require careful planning and organisation of every stage in their conduct. Research subjects have to be found and booked in at appropriate times and the experimental conditions need to be carefully established and monitored. In experiments, attempts are always made to control or at least measure the influence of as many variables as possible whilst altering only the independent variable (IV) of interest. The effect of the independent variable on the outcome measure which is the the dependent variable (DV) can be best determined when all other variables are held constant. These extraneous variables might include, for example, ambient temperature or background noise depending upon the nature of the investigation.

Like all research, initial steps in designing an experiment depend upon the clarity of the definition of the problem and questions being investigated. The design of the study may use a combination of independent groups, that is, different groups of research subjects, and repeated measures using each subject as their own control. The reasoning and the questions being asked will help determine the design of the experiment. It is not usually desirable, however, in student project work, to investigate all aspects of a piece of research in one all-embracing experimental design. Such complex designs are frequently problematical to analyse and interpret properly. In most cases, it is better to break down the study into a number of discrete experiments, each investigating a specific aspect of the phenomena under consideration.

The variable being changed in an experiment is the independent variable (IV). It could be the concentrations of a substance being investigated, which is a direct alteration of an independent variable. In many experiments, however, the experimenter is making use of naturally occuring variations – such as the existence of female and male genders – to manipulate these independent variables by their allocation to particular groups. The effects of a number of different independent variables may be investigated within the same experimental situation, although as has been pointed out earlier, the analyses of these designs can become complex. The values of the independent variable are frequently called the 'conditions' in psychological experiments and are referred to as the 'factor levels' in statistical analysis.

The variable which is being recorded in some way as the outcome measure in an experiment is thus the dependent variable (DV). More than one dependent variable may be recorded in an experiment, and if these are to be analysed together, particularly sophisticated analyses known as multivariate statistical techniques are required, which are beyond the scope of introductory statistics and of many student projects.

Lab work requires a good deal of discipline and organisation on the part of the researcher if the results are to be repeatable and meaningful. Much of the time, you will be doing the same thing over and over again. You may be measuring the levels of a substance in the blood of research subjects and may need to run the analysis under different experimental conditions for many different research subjects, keeping the environment or other conditions as constant as possible. You are likely to be using published procedures, or protocols, for the biochemical analysis and possibly for the experimental procedures. A bugbear for many lab workers is not being able to reproduce published findings, often as a starting point for their own experiments. Sometimes this arises because the methods section of the published paper may omit some critical details of the way the experiment or the analysis was conducted. Sometimes even apparantly trivial details of method, such as the source of the chemicals, which might affect the purity, can be crucial. Many potentially promising laboratory investigations have become bogged down in such methodological problems.

One lesson from this is to try to ensure that your own results are replicable. This might mean, in practice, recording every detail of what you have done and writing these up in your report or paper reporting the findings. You need to be slightly obsessive in adhering strictly to protocols and ensuring consistency each time the experiment is run. Many lab procedures are now automated, so that computer-controlled machines and biochemical autoanalysers are commonplace. These can free the researcher from the need to attend to many procedures which need to be held constant, but before relying upon them, any such equipment which you may wish to use needs to be checked out. The calibration of equipment needs to be checked and set prior to its deployment. Even if other people have been using the equipment for a similar purpose, you should always check the calibration.

Calibration often involves running certain standard conditions and checking the output against expected results. The reliability or reproducibility of data can also be checked in this way, for example by running the same concentrations of samples through machines on different occasions. These procedures also enable you to gain an estimate of the likely error in your measurements. Thus, for example, a procedure may produce an average agreement of duplicate samples of, say, 5 or 10 per cent. Any attempt to measure changes caused by the manipulation of the independent variable in your research subjects which are not expected to be at least as large as this is therefore not going to succeed.

The outcome of many experiments is therefore inconclusive because the variability in the experimental results swamps the effects that you may be trying to measure. Ways of minimising the effects of such variability centre on increasing the sample size, increasing the degree of control over the independent variables and improving the experimental design and methodological procedures. Once you are satisfied, however, that equipment and conditions have been optimally set, you are ready to run your experiments.

Remember that when research subjects are being brought into the laboratory, they may find it a strange or even a hostile or intimidating place. The subjects may not behave in a typical manner, that is, the laboratory may not provide ecologically valid data. This is particularly salient for some social and psychological investigations. Familiarisation and 'settling down' procedures may need to be allowed for. In many experimental investigations, it may be possible to use freely available volunteers without the need, as in survey research, to go to great lengths to find representative or random samples of the population of interest. This is because laboratory investigations such as estimates of back strength or blood biochemistry or visual acuity or some other basic physiological or psychological variable are, as a rule, more generalisable than data, for example, concerning attitudes or behaviour using a survey methodology. Consequently, many laboratory investigations rely on volunteers amongst the student population. However, the degree to which this group may provide a valid sample needs to be carefully thought about in the design of an experiment.

It is also true, as a rule of thumb, that laboratory investigations may be conducted with smaller sample sizes than are required, for example, for a survey. Thus, with an appropriate balanced design, as few as sixteen or twenty experimental subjects may be sufficient to produce reliable and statistically sound findings. Indeed, it has been argued that if experiments require large samples for the detection of effects you may not be dealing with 'robust' data, in the sense that there may not be clear-cut differences related to the conditions of the independent variable. However, this is a generalisation which clearly depends on the design of the study, the amount of variability in the experimental procedures and so on. Some of the most challenging and innovative experimental work is often concerned with establishing the right conditions to be able to detect effects against a background of variability and unwanted effects of independent variables.

Designs for experimental laboratory work may be of several different types, with the following as typical. Repeated measures designs are frequently used, whereby multiple measurements are taken at various points on the same research subjects. Using subjects as their own controls in this way is economical of research subjects, but is clearly not always practicable. For example, it is not possible to use a repeated measures design where the influence of earlier measurements may seriously affect the later ones. An alternative is to use either matched subjects or independent groups. A matched pairs design involves pairing each person in the experimental group with one in the control group. The pairing may be carried out on one or more relevant variables such as age, gender, psychomotor ability or whatever is of relevance to the study. Once the pairing has been carried out, the subjects in each pair are then randomly allocated to either an experimental or a control group.

Independent groups designs involve allocating subjects into two or more separate groups, usually by a process of randomisation. The principal disadvantages of this design are that differences in the dependent variable may be attributable to differences between the groups as well as differences in the effects of the independent variable, and greater numbers of subjects need to be recruited compared to the repeated measures designs.

Experimental studies, therefore, normally involve two or more different conditions. Clearly, if the various conditions are presented in the same sequence each time, there is the possibility of distortion or bias due to order effects. For example, the effects of the first condition may alter the subjects' responses to subsequent experimental conditions. In order to deal with order effects, counterbalancing may be employed. Thus, if there were two conditions, half of the subjects would experience condition A first and then condition B, while the other half would have the sequence reversed. More complex counterbalancing is possible. Randomisation of conditions, where there may be a large number of experimental conditions, is another possibility.

Once the design of the experiment has been established, normally after some pilot work has been carried out on the feasibility of the methods to be employed, the data can be collected. It is important that a standard and systematised procedure is adhered to, whatever type of experiment it may be. Thus instructions to subjects involved in the experiment should be given either in written form or, if verbal, these should be repeated verbatim for each subject. A lab notebook should be kept, which provides the written protocol for the experiment. A note of the order in which things are carried out, instructions for making up the reagents, machine settings and so on, should all be documented in the notebook. The results need to be kept in the notebook as they are obtained, together with associated machine printouts and so on.

Experimenter expectancy effects, that is, expectations about the outcome of an experiment, can exert a subtle influence which can operate at an entirely unconscious level. Cues given to

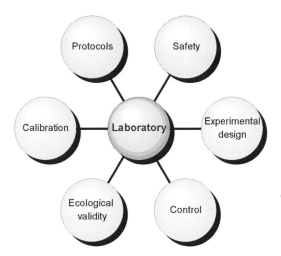

Figure 6.1   Key issues in conducting a laboratory study.

subjects can be influenced by tone of voice, experimenter attitudes and a host of other factors. Wherever possible, therefore, the experiment should be conducted 'blind', that is, without knowledge to which condition subjects have been allocated. If this is not possible, then at the least the processing of the resulting data can be carried out blind by such techniques as the allocation of codes to experimental conditions.

Finally, do not forget the importance of debriefing people, that is, fully explaining the purpose and outcome of the study to those who have been helpful enough to take part in your experiments. Even if it was not possible fully to inform the subjects about the purpose of the experiment at the outset, as in some psychological experiments, for example, they should at least be debriefed on completion. People generally do not like to feel they are being used by researchers as 'guinea pigs' and should be treated as human beings. Valuable feedback can often be obtained by discussing the experiment with subjects afterwards, and people are generally interested in knowing more about the research.

Underlying all laboratory work is the need to pay particular attention to safety issues, including the wearing of laboratory coats and safety equipment such as rubber gloves and eye protection where required. This goes without saying where dangerous or hazardous substances are being handled, as in biochemical laboratories, but applies more generally in any laboratory setting. Psychological laboratories, for example, often make use of electrical recording equipment which can be hazardous to research subjects if not carefully handled and maintained. Exercise testing and other physiological investigations may be hazardous to the subjects if agreed protocols are not strictly adhered to. For all of these reasons, student research projects being carried out in the laboratory are always conducted under expert supervision. It is important for the researcher to make sure that approved protocols are adhered to and that there are agreed procedures to be followed should things go wrong. It is also the responsibility of the researcher to be aware of the relevant regulations governing laboratory investigations such as the COSHH (Control of Substances Hazardous to Health) regulations and specific regulations controlling, for example, microbiological, virological and radioisotope investigations. Figure 6.1 summarises some of the key issues in conducting laboratory experimental work that have been introduced.

Action points

- Carefully plan your laboratory study, taking into account the facilities available.
- Carefully choose the appropriate research design.
- Conduct a pilot study to determine the size of expected effects and test methods.
- Use an appropriate statistical analysis based upon the research design which has been employed.

Chapter 7

Getting to grips with stats

It is hard to get very far without numbers, yet numerical concepts can cause many people difficulty, especially those who may have been away from formal schooling for some years and have forgotten much of what was learned in mathematics classes. This chapter is meant as a primer and is concerned with introducing some numerical and statistical concepts developed further in the next chapter.

What is the statistical method?

The statistical method is concerned with the collection, analysis and interpretation of numerical data. The discipline of applied statistics is frequently divided into descriptive statistics and inferential statistics. The former is concerned with describing data and centres on the presentation of numbers in such forms as summary tables and charts. The calculation of measures of average and measures of dispersion, or variability, of the data is in the realm of descriptive statistics. Inferential statistics, on the other hand, are concerned with drawing conclusions about the data, for example by determining whether the means of two or more sets of numbers differ by a degree which cannot reasonably be attributed to chance variation; that is, they are statistically 'significantly different'. Unfortunately, the discipline of statistics has a bad name in some quarters which is epitomised by the well known saying of Benjamin Disraeli, 'There are lies, damned lies and statistics'. However, this should serve as encouragement to get to grips with the subject since only by appreciating the ways in which data and analytical techniques can be misused will you be in a position to form an opinion on the reliability or otherwise of figures with which you are presented.

Data can be used for purposes for which it was never originally collected or intended, the collection process can be flawed and the analytical process can also be flawed. Data can be presented in a biased or misleading way by such means as the use of charts where the vertical scale does not start at zero, thereby visually exaggerating the size of differences between points on the chart. Figures 7.1 and 7.2 represent exactly the same data from an experimental study. This study was concerned with the measurement of brain electrical activity following nerve stimulation at various frequencies ranging from 1Hz to 500Hz. In Figure 7.1, the vertical axis represents only a small part of the range shown in Figure 7.2 and the researchers wished to argue that a cyclical frequency-dependent pattern of responses was observed. Figure 7.2, however, emphasises that the values of the responses at each frequency were very similar, and that the percentage changes were extremely small. A statistical analysis would, in practice, be necessary to determine whether these fluctuations were, or were not, of the order to be expected by chance; the point emphasised here is that visually the impact of the two ways of presenting the same observations in these charts is very different.

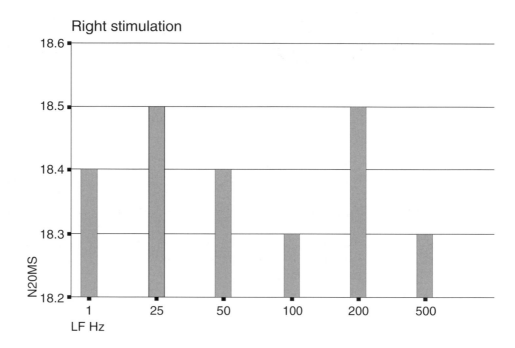

Figure 7.1 Data from measurement of brain electrical activity with vertical scale starting at non-zero. The same data is presented in Figure 7.2.

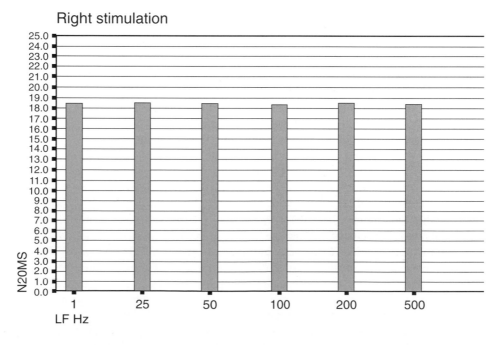

Figure 7.2 Data from measurement of brain electrical activity with vertical scale starting at zero.

These types of problems of interpretation may be encountered when dealing with secondary data, that is, data which other people have collected and presented. Other difficulties with such data sources are that the data may not be relevant or up-to-date, we may not have much information on how the data was collected and analysed, and complete data may not be available for our purposes. It is advisable to treat any such secondary data with a healthy scepticism until these points have been clarified, and always to remember that just because something has been published in a scientific journal, this does not guarantee its validity or accuracy.

Everyone is familiar with the pie chart as is shown in Figure 8.5. The pie chart represents a very simple level of describing data; the chart indicates what percentage of the total of 100 per cent is represented by the different categories of which it is comprised. The pie chart is an example of a univariate analysis, that is, presenting and analysing information related to a single variable. A variable is anything which can vary or take different values, such as gender (the values male and female), social class or height. In practice, much data analysis is concerned with examining more than a single variable. Examining two variables in relation to each other is the area of bivariate analysis; for example, taller people tend to be heavier, so there is a correlation, or association, of the two variables. Examining differences between two groups is another example of a bivariate analysis; for example, are the average heights of men and women different? When statisticians address this question, they are actually asking a particular technical question: 'Are the differences in the measured heights of a sample of men and women the sort of variations that could reasonably be attributed to chance factors or is there is real, statistically significant difference in the average heights?' Statisticians, therefore, deal with probabilities, or the balance of evidence, rather than certainties. By convention, if something is likely to have occurred less than 1 in 20 times purely by chance, statisticians will feel entitled to reject chance as the explanation and accept instead that there is another explanation accounting for the association or the difference. This is expressed statistically as $P < 0.05$, that is, the probability of occurrence by chance is less than 5 out of 100.

Statistics also deals with more complex data analysis problems in practice; if the differences or associations between three or more variables are being examined, then multivariate statistical procedures apply. For example, if we were to require a statistical answer to the question 'Do the average heights of men and women influence their choice of occupation?', assuming we had collected data on the variables gender, height and occupation, we would require multivariate statistical techniques.

Different sorts of numbers

Numbers can, of course, come in many forms. The numbers on the shirts of a football team are there by convention only and have no mathematical significance – this is called a nominal scale or categorical variable. Another example of a nominal scale item would be the numeric codes assigned to questionnaire items such as the following.

| No | 0 |
| Yes | 1 |

A further example would be numbers coding for gender in a spreadsheet. In each of these cases, the numbers are merely labels and these could easily be transposed without any effect on subsequent statistical analysis.

Another type of number, or level of measurement, is represented by the following question-naire examples.

The doctors at the surgery listen to me.

5	4	3	2	1
Strongly agree	Agree	Undecided	Disagree	Strongly disagree

Please indicate your age group by circling a number from the list below:

16–25 years	1
26–35 years	2
36–45 years	3
46–55 years	4
56–65 years	5
Over 65 years	6

These are both examples of ordinal scale items. The characteristic of an ordinal scale is that the *direction* of the numbers is meaningful, unlike nominal scale items. Thus it is sensible to assign adjacent numeric codes to the 5 point scale item above, since the direction of the con-cept of agreement matches up with the direction of the numbers. What is not mathematically meaningful, however, is the *size* of the differences in the numbers – it is not conceptually sen-sible, for example, to argue that the difference between Strongly agree and Agree is the same as the difference between Agree and Undecided. Because of this characteristic, statistical analyses which can be used with ordinal scale items work on the rank ordering of the numbers and not their absolute differences.

Other levels of measurement are interval scales and ratio scales. These share all of the prop-erties of ordinal scales and, in addition, here the size of the differences in the numbers becomes meaningful. Height and weight are examples of ratio scales, so that a person weigh-ing 140 kg is exactly twice as heavy as one weighing 70 kg and so forth. A ratio scale also has an absolute zero point as a reference point; the importance of this is that ratios (such as 140:70 in the above example) are appropriate since there is the reference of an absolute zero, whereas with interval scales there are equal intervals across the whole range of numbers employed, but the zero is an arbitrary one. An example of an equal interval scale is the Celsius temperature scale where the zero is the freezing point of water, but negative temperatures are possible. It is not possible to say, therefore, with this temperature scale that 20 degrees is twice the tempera-ture of 10 degrees. Many statistical tests demand at least an interval scale level of measure-ment as an assumption for their appropriate application.

The normal distribution

Some numbers, such as the number of children in a family, can only exist as whole integers: these are discrete variables. Other numbers represent continuous variables which can be

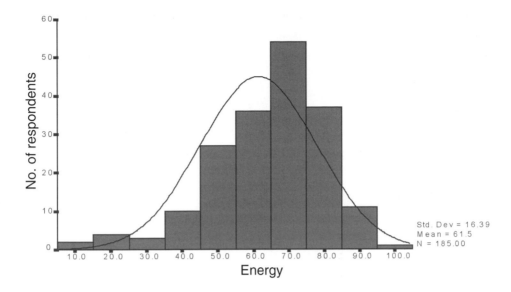

Figure 7.3   Histogram of data from an analogue rating scale questionnaire item where respondents were asked to rate their energy levels on a scale of 0–100. An acceptably normal distribution has been obtained for the purposes of statistical testing. The curved line represents a true normal distribution.

measured to a greater and greater precision depending on the measuring instrument, such as the weight or the height of people in a sample drawn from a population.

If the heights of a sample of a hundred 100 people were measured in this way and plotted on a chart where the horizontal axis (the *x* axis) was marked in metres and the vertical axis (the *y* axis) represented the number of individuals at each height, a curve would be produced by joining up all the points representing the heights of each individual. Most people are going to be around 'average' height and the number of very short and very tall people will be much smaller. The curve will therefore exhibit a hump in the middle, gradually dropping off at each side. Plotting data in this way produces a frequency distribution. A histogram is an alternative way of presenting such data, and consists of a series of bars where the height of each bar represents the number of individuals falling into a particular range of values, or class interval.

A special type of frequency distribution is called the normal distribution which is a symmetrical 'bell-shaped' curve. Many statistical tests make assumptions about the population characteristics or parameters, that is, they rest on an assumption about the normality of the underlying distribution of the population data and these tests are called parametric tests. The use of the term normal to describe such a distribution is a technical one and it has no implications for the usual or the expected distribution of a set of data. An example of an approximately normal distribution is illustrated in Figure 7.3. The histogram illustrates the data from a sample of 185 survey respondents who rated their energy levels. A normal curve has been superimposed upon it. This data is showing a slight negative skew, that is, there is a tail towards the low end values, but would be regarded as acceptably normal for the purposes of parametric testing.

On the other hand, an example of a data distribution which is very far from normal is

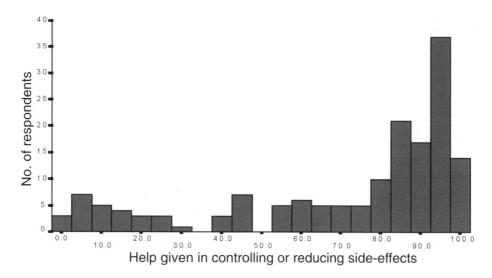

No. of respondents

Help given in controlling or reducing side-effects

Figure 7.4   Histogram of data from an analogue rating scale questionnaire item on helpfulness of staff on a scale of 0–100. The data indicates a strong skew towards the upper end of the range (80–100) and would not be suitable for analysis by parametric statistical tests.

illustrated in Figure 7.4. This illustrates the highly skewed responses from an analogue scale questionnaire item obtained from a sample of patients who rated, on a scale of 0–100, the help they had been given by ward staff in controlling the side effects of chemotherapy medication. The histogram indicates that most people felt they had been given a great deal of help, with the bulk of responses falling in the 80–100 range.

In practice, data is rarely perfect in forming a normally distributed shape, and fortunately, many statistical tests which rest on the assumption of normality of a population are robust enough to allow for deviations. Many distributions are skewed in one direction or the other. A positively skewed distribution has a long 'tail' which veers off to the high values (the right-hand part of the curve) whilst a negatively skewed distribution has a tail veering to the low values, representing more observations at these data values than would be expected in a normal distribution.

Descriptive statistics

A normal or near normal distribution can be described by a measure of average, usually the arithmetic mean, and by a measure of variability or spread of the data. The mean is calculated by adding up all the observations in the dataset and dividing by the total number. The measure of variability which is commonly used is called the standard deviation. Just over 68 per cent of all the cases will fall within one standard deviation on either side of the mean of a normal distribution, and approximately 95 per cent will fall within a range two standard deviations on either side of the mean. The larger the size of the standard deviation, the greater the spread or dispersion of the scores; the standard deviation is used in preference to the range (the difference between the highest and lowest scores) since the range is sensitive to extreme or outlying values in a way that the standard deviation is not. The smaller the standard deviation, the more the scores will be concentrated around the mean, producing a highly peaked curve. This type of curve is called leptokurtic and is contrasted with a widely dispersed or flatter curve which is called platykurtic. A mesokurtic shape falls between these two extremes. The standard deviation is calculated by:

- finding the overall mean of the data
- finding the deviation of each reading from the overall mean
- squaring these deviations
- adding up all the squared deviations
- dividing this sum by the total number of readings
- taking the square root of the resulting sum.

When data that has been collected is subject to a severe skew, which can be visually determined, for example, by plotting the points as a histogram (see Figure 7.3), the arithmetic mean and the standard deviation are not the descriptive statistics of choice. The median provides a better measure of average in such situations. The median, also called the fiftieth percentile, is that value up to which 50 per cent of all the cases lie when they are arranged in order. That is, it is the middle value if there is an unequal number of cases, or halfway between the two middle values if there is an equal number of cases. The other measure of average which is sometimes encountered is the mode – which is the most frequently occurring value in the data. Instead of the standard deviation, in order to describe the dispersion of highly skewed data, the semi-interquartile range may be used. The semi-interquartile range is calculated by taking half the difference between the middle 50 per cent of the data. The median and the semi-interquartile range are relatively insensitive to the large group of extreme values accounting for the skew in the distribution, compared to the mean and standard deviation. In a normal distribution, the three measures of average, that is, the mean, the median and the mode, all have precisely the same value.

Inferential statistics

Much of statistical analysis is concerned with comparing data against certain expectations and making a decision about the differences. This is the area of inferential statistical analysis. If the differences between the data and the expected could not reasonably be attributed to chance, the differences are termed statistically significant. Formally speaking, a null hypothesis and an alternative or research hypothesis are set up and the results of statistical testing employed to reach a decision about which is correct, at a certain degree of probability. Thus statistics cannot unequivocally rule out chance as an explanation for findings but only render it sufficiently implausible for chance to be accepted as a reasonable explanation of findings. By statistical convention, if findings could have arisen by chance less than 5 per cent of the time, chance may be rejected as an explanation.

There are two types of error which can be made in arriving at a decision as to whether to accept or reject the null hypothesis. Statisticians call the first error a Type I error which involves rejecting the null hypothesis when, in fact, the null hypothesis is true. A Type II error, on the other hand, implies accepting the null hypothesis when it is false. The ability to achieve a balance between making the two types of error brings in the idea of the power of a statistical test. The power of a test reflects the probability of rejecting the null hypothesis when it is, in fact, false. The most powerful tests are generally those which make a number of assumptions about the normality, the variabilities and the scales of measurement of the data from the associated populations. Generally speaking, the power of a statistical test also increases as the sample size increases.

The null hypothesis means you are assuming 'no effects' by default and, for example, assumes no differences between the means of groups, other than random errors arising by chance, whereas the alternative hypothesis is stating that the means are not equal. If the alternative hypothesis is stated in this way, it is called a two-tailed hypothesis, that is, the mean of one group could be either statistically significantly larger or smaller than the mean of another group. The test for one mean being significantly only larger than the other would be a one-tailed test, and similarly, if the test were that the mean of one group was predicted to be significantly smaller than the other. Normally, two-tailed tests of significance are employed in most studies, since there is usually no good evidence that the difference in, say, an experimental group is only likely to arise in one direction. This is an important point; in practice, the probability levels for one-tailed testing are half the values appropriate to two-tailed testing and data can therefore be 'statistically significant' when a one-tailed test is used whereas the data might not be if a two-tailed test were to be used.

Inferential statistics, as we have seen, typically demands certain characteristics of the populations from which the sample data was drawn. An assumption of normal distribution is common, as is an assumption that two sets of data were drawn from populations having an equal spread of scores, that is, variances. If these assumptions cannot reasonably be expected to be true, and there are recognised ways of assessing these, the use of alternative inferential statistical tests may be available which do not require these assumptions. This latter group is called non-parametric or distribution free tests. These points are picked up in the next chapter which provides examples of data analysed with each type of test.

Action points

- Examine the data collected and take advice concerning its analysis.
- Decide on analyses appropriate to the levels of measurement and the purposes of the study.

Chapter 8

Not everything that counts ...

If your project involves the collection of numerical information, perhaps from an experimental investigation or from a closed questionnaire, you will normally wish to enter the data on a computer and provide a statistical analysis. Suitable packages for entering data include databases, spreadsheets and statistical analysis packages such as SPSS (Statistical Package for the Social Sciences). The production of charts from your data can also be accomplished using statistical and spreadsheet packages.

The questions asked in the research and the design of the study will imply certain ways of analysing the ensuing data. As has been made clear in earlier chapters, for experimental studies where several groups are involved and perhaps multiple measurements taken, designs can become quite complex, making the subsequent task of data analysis less than straightforward. You are advised as novice researchers to choose the most straightforward design which is sufficient to address the question of interest. This may mean taking decisions early on not to include measurements of some variables, although in your report you will need to justify the approach you eventually adopt.

Entering data

Your data needs to be entered in the appropriate form for the statistical analysis which you have in mind, whatever package you use to enter the data. Thus each column in a database table or spreadsheet normally contains the values for one variable, such as one question on a questionnaire, and each row becomes one case. There should not be any blank rows in your block of data, even though spreadsheets will allow this facility in order to improve the layout, as these will be treated as missing data by the statistical analysis package. Sometimes questionnaires contain questions where more than one response may be selected for a particular question, that is, the response options are not mutually exclusive. Where this is the case, one column is set up for *each item* in the list of options, and an appropriate value (such as 1) is entered if that item is selected and another value (such as zero) is entered if it is not. Similarly, the handling of lists of items ranked in order of importance or preference will be treated in an analogous way. A separate column is set up for each and the rank order assigned to that item is then entered in each column. An example of this data entry format is shown in Figure 8.1. This data was entered in Microsoft Excel. Blank cells represent data that is missing. The variable names appear on the first row – these should be kept short and should not contain any spaces, but can contain the underscore character (_) if the data is subsequently to be imported and analysed using a statistical analysis package like SPSS. In this example, which is data collected on waiting times in child health clinics, some variables have been set up as date variables and

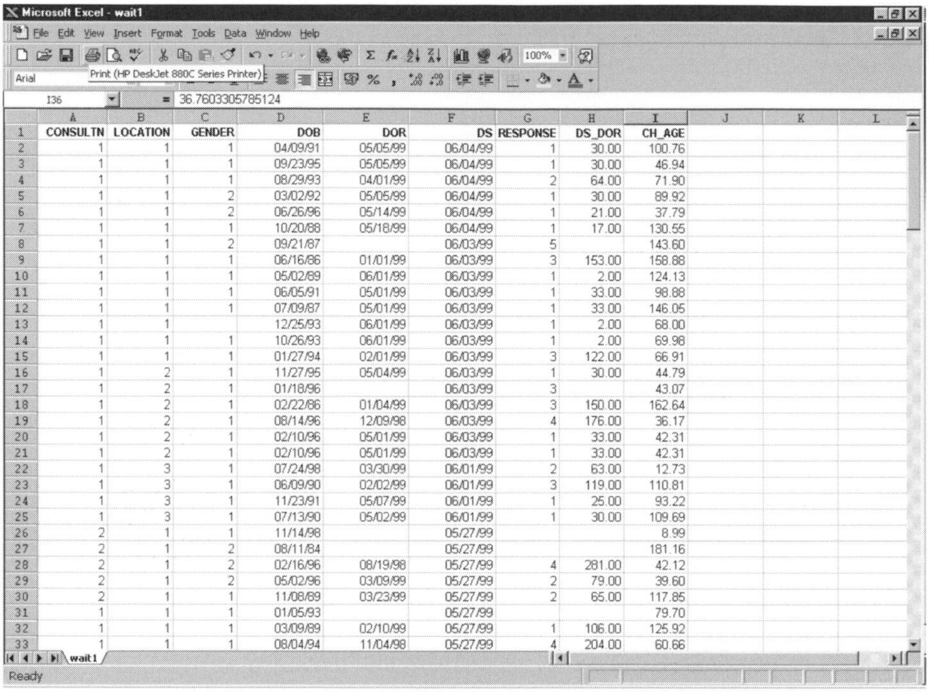

	A	B	C	D	E	F	G	H	I	J	K	L
1	CONSULTN	LOCATION	GENDER	DOB	DOR	DS	RESPONSE	DS_DOR	CH_AGE			
2	1	1	1	04/09/91	05/05/99	06/04/99	1	30.00	100.76			
3	1	1	1	09/23/95	05/05/99	06/04/99	1	30.00	46.94			
4	1	1	1	08/29/93	04/01/99	06/04/99	2	64.00	71.90			
5	1	1	2	03/02/92	05/05/99	06/04/99	1	30.00	89.92			
6	1	1	2	06/26/96	05/14/99	06/04/99	1	21.00	37.79			
7	1	1	1	10/20/88	05/18/99	06/04/99	1	17.00	130.55			
8	1	1	2	09/21/87		06/03/99	5		143.60			
9	1	1	1	06/16/86	01/01/99	06/03/99	3	153.00	158.88			
10	1	1	1	05/02/89	06/01/99	06/03/99	1	2.00	124.13			
11	1	1	1	06/05/91	05/01/99	06/03/99	1	33.00	98.88			
12	1	1	1	07/09/87	05/01/99	06/03/99	1	33.00	146.05			
13	1	1		12/25/93	06/01/99	06/03/99	1	2.00	68.00			
14	1	1	1	10/26/93	06/01/99	06/03/99	1	2.00	69.98			
15	1	1	1	01/27/94	02/01/99	06/03/99	3	122.00	66.91			
16	1	2	1	11/27/95	05/04/99	06/03/99	1	30.00	44.79			
17	1	2	1	01/18/96		06/03/99	3		43.07			
18	1	2	1	02/22/86	01/04/99	06/03/99	3	150.00	162.64			
19	1	2	1	08/14/96	12/09/98	06/03/99	4	176.00	36.17			
20	1	2	1	02/10/96	05/01/99	06/03/99	1	33.00	42.31			
21	1	2	1	02/10/96	05/01/99	06/03/99	1	33.00	42.31			
22	1	3	1	07/24/98	03/30/99	06/01/99	2	63.00	12.73			
23	1	3	1	06/09/90	02/02/99	06/01/99	3	119.00	110.81			
24	1	3	1	11/23/91	05/07/99	06/01/99	1	25.00	93.22			
25	1	3	1	07/13/90	05/02/99	06/01/99	1	30.00	109.69			
26	2	1	1	11/14/98		05/27/99			8.99			
27	2	1	2	08/11/84		05/27/99			181.16			
28	2	1	2	02/16/96	08/19/98	05/27/99	4	281.00	42.12			
29	2	1	2	05/02/96	03/09/99	05/27/99	2	79.00	39.60			
30	2	1	1	11/08/89	03/23/99	05/27/99	2	65.00	117.85			
31	1	1	1	01/05/93		05/27/99			79.70			
32	1	1	1	03/09/89	02/10/99	05/27/99	1	106.00	125.92			
33	1	1	1	08/04/94	11/04/98	05/27/99	4	204.00	60.66			

Figure 8.1   Screenshot of data in Microsoft Excel.

entered in a standard way (DD/MM/YY) and others are numeric variables entered either as whole digits or as integers and decimal places.

As a general rule, data should be entered onto a computer in the most detailed or precise form in which it has been collected and it should not usually be summarised or rounded in any way, since rounding is the final stage of an analysis. This is because you can instruct statistical software to group and summarise the data in the most appropriate ways depending upon the results of preliminary exploratory analyses. Thus, for example, if age in years has been recorded it should be entered as exact age rather than summarised into age groups. If you enter summary data, you are likely to find that you have lost flexibility at a later stage. There are exceptions to this general rule, however. For example, you may have collected data using a standard psychological or social questionnaire and it may not actually be necessary to enter all the individual scores item by item. This situation could arise if you are confining your analysis to scores calculated for particular dimensions composed of weighted or unweighted summaries across a number of items. It may, in fact, save some time and effort to calculate the dimension scores on each questionnaire beforehand using mental arithmetic and only to enter the required summary information.

Analysing data from nominal scales

Figure 8.2 provides an overall conceptual scheme for the various analyses discussed here. It needs to be said at the outset that there are many more statistical procedures available to the data analyst but many of these are highly specialised or require particular expertise in their use

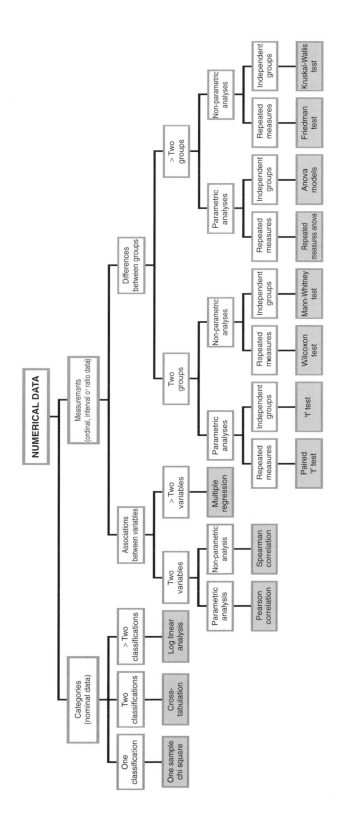

Figure 8.2 A statistical decision-making chart.

Table 8.1   Table of frequencies from two survey questionnaire items

Gender of respondent

		Frequency	Per cent	Valid %	Cumulative %
Valid	Female	72	45.0	45.0	45.0
	Male	88	55.0	55.0	100.0
	Total	160	100.0	100.0	
Total		160	100.0		

Whether registered with GP

		Frequency	Per cent	Valid %	Cumulative %
Valid	No	26.0	16.3	16.3	16.3
	No	122.0	76.3	76.3	92.5
Unsure		12	7.5	7.5	100.0
	Total	160.0	100.0	100.0	

or interpretation, which is beyond the scope of this book. Working from the top of the tree in Figure 8.2, you may have numerical data either in the form of categories, that is, nominal scale items as have been introduced in the previous chapter, or the data may be in the form of measurements. Let us take categorical data first.

If you have carried out a survey using a closed questionnaire, you are likely to have a combination of nominal and ordinal scale items to analyse, although some variables, such as age, may also be measured at the ratio level. Let us say you had a number of items which were of the following type:

Please indicate your gender

Female	0
Male	1

Are you registered with a GP?

No	0
Yes	1
Unsure	2

These are both nominal scale items and your analysis is likely to concentrate on first producing frequency counts for each variable, that is, the number and percentage in the sample who answered each option for each of these items. Frequency tables produced by the SPSS statistical software for these variables, which were included in a survey of 160 first year health studies students, are shown in Table 8.1.

In each case the tables show the category, the number (frequency) and percentages of the sample of 160 represented by each category. In the above tables, the column marked 'valid per cent' is the same as the per cent; if there were any missing data, the valid per cent column would exclude the missing cases.

Further analysis that is possible with nominal scale items includes examining relationships between variables; in the above example, you might be interested in determining whether there is an association between gender of respondents and the way they have answered the question. You can use the cross-tabulation procedure to classify the values of one nominal variable against another. The SPSS output from a cross-tabulation of these variables from the student survey is shown in Table 8.2.

In the first part of Table 8.2, there are three values in each of the six cells in the table. The topmost value in each cell represents the number, also known as the observed frequencies, of males and females who answered each option. The middle figure in each cell represents the expected frequencies, that is, the numbers expected if there was no association between gender and the responses to the question. Finally, the bottom row in each cell is the percentage of males and females who answered each option. The table shows, therefore, that about 85 per cent of the female students were registered with a GP whereas the comparable figure for the males was about 69 per cent. Is there a statistically significant association between gender and the pattern of responses obtained to the question?

The chi-square test can be applied to determine whether there is a relationship between the variables. In the above example, the calculated chi-square statistic was 6.34 and this was statistically significant ($p < 0.05$ – actually equal to 0.042 in the above example). A problem which may be encountered with this analysis is that, as a widely used rule of thumb, no more than 20 per cent of the cells in such a table (which in the above 2×3 table would be no more than one cell) should have expected values less than 5, and no cell should have expected values less than 1. It is the not the numbers, i.e. observed values, that should adhere to this rule, but the expected values which the statistics package will calculate and which can be displayed in the table. Thus, if there is a small sample, and very few people answered the 'unsure' option, this problem may be encountered. One way round this difficulty is to combine categories of responses into larger categories. An alternative analysis to the chi-square test for tables where there are two rows and two columns, which is not affected by the small cell expected frequencies problem, is the Fisher's exact test which is automatically computed by the SPSS software for 2×2 tables when one or more cells have expected frequencies under 5.

Alongside the value of the test statistic, the output from a computerised statistical analysis will include the associated probability and will also include a figure known as degrees of freedom (DF), as is shown in the table above. The degrees of freedom are normally calculated by taking the sample size and subtracting one or more values, depending upon the nature of the analysis. The degrees of freedom may be calculated therefore as $n - 1$ or $n - 2$ (or some other value) as appropriate. The degrees of freedom should be stated when you are presenting the results of a statistical analysis. In the cross-tabulation example shown above, the degrees of freedom are equal to the number of rows minus 1, multiplied by the number of columns minus 1 – that is, 2 in this example.

Table 8.2 The computer output from the cross-tabulation procedure using the chi-square test of independence

Whether registered with GP — Gender of respondent cross-tablulation

			Gender of respondent		
			Female	Male	Total
Whether registered with GP	No	Count	6	20	26
		Expected count	11.7	14.3	26.0
		per cent within gender of respondent	8.3	22.7	16.3
	Yes	Count	61	61	122
		Expected count	54.9	67.1	122.0
		per cent within gender of respondent	84.7	69.3	76.3
	Unsure	Count	5	7	12
		Expected count	5.4	6.6	12.0
		per cent within gender of respondent	6.9	8.0	7.5
		Count	72	88	160
		Expected count	72.0	88.0	160.0
		per cent within gender of respondent	100.0	100.0	100.0

Chi-square tests

	Value	df	Asymp. sig. (2 sided)
Pearson Chi-Square	6.335[a]	2	0.042
Likelihood ratio	6.685	2	0.035
Linear-by-linear association		1	0.080
No. of valid classes	160		

Note: [a] 0 cells (0.0%) have expected count less than 5. The minimum expected count is 5.40.

Analysing data from ordinal scales

Many questionnaire items use an ordinal scale: for example, attitudinal items as below:

Health promotion is an important part of my work.

Strongly Agree	Unsure	Disagree	Strongly Agreee	Disagree
1	2	3	4	5

Once again, frequency counts can be applied to determine the number of overall responses made at each scale point. You can, however, go further with ordinal scale items and apply a range of non-parametric tests. See Figure 8.2 again: with ordinal scale items we have genuine measurements of some variables. You may be interested in either measuring the extent of association between the variables, in which case the non-parametric correlation coefficient (Spearman rank correlation) may be used. On the other hand, or in addition, you may be interested in determining whether two or more groups are statistically significantly different in their medians. The various statistical tests listed in Figure 8.2 under non-parametric analyses are appropriate here. Thus, if you wish to determine whether the males and females in the sample significantly differed in their responses to these items, you could use the Mann–Whitney test, which is appropriate for ordinal variables when there are two independent groups. Another example of the use of the Mann–Whitney test is shown next.

The Mann–Whitney test

A nurse administered an eleven point pain rating scale where patients were asked to indicate, on a scale ranging from 0 (no pain) to 10 (as intense as imaginable), their level of pain following surgery. Eighteen patients were studied and 10 were assigned to receive fixed doses of an analgesic. Eight patients were given a patient controlled analgesia (PCA) device. The data was as follows:

PCA group	Fixed dose group
5	9
5	8
4	4
3	7
6	5
7	5
5	8
3	6
	7
	5

A Mann–Whitney test indicated that the mean rank of the fixed dose group was 11.65 and of the PCA group was 6.81. This indicates that the PCA group tended more often to choose options towards the lower end (less pain) of the scale. The normal approximation to the Mann–Whitney test statistic indicated a z value of 1.95 with an associated probability of 0.051. The null hypothesis that there were no differences between the groups in the amount of pain experienced was therefore retained. The data is very marginal, however, and suggests a strong trend to a more favourable outcome in the PCA group. An independent samples t test indicates that the means of the two groups are statistically significantly different ($t = 2.26$, DF= 16, $P< 0.05$) and reveals the greater power of parametric tests which use all of the information about the size of differences.

Another non-parametric test suitable for the analysis of ordinal scale items is the Wilcoxon test. This is a repeated measures test, that is, it is suitable when there are two sets of measurements made on the same group of subjects. An example of its use is shown next.

The Wilcoxon paired-sample test

A sociologist was interested in assessing the immediate impact of a talk on healthy lifestyles on the attitudes of a group of adolescents. A group of 12 young people was recruited and was asked to rate their attitudes towards a statement on a topic of interest, using a 7 point scale ranging from 1 (Completely agree) to 7 (Completely disagree), just prior to and just after listening to the talk. The following data was obtained.

Subject	Before	After
1	2	3
2	3	5
3	3	3
4	3	6
5	5	6
6	6	5
7	4	5
8	3	4
9	5	6
10	4	5
11	2	4
12	3	4

The Wilcoxon paired samples test calculates the ranks of the differences between the before and after measurements for this data. The data indicates that in 10 subjects there had been a shift towards a higher scale point (that is, more disagreement with the statement); in one subject the shift was in the opposite direction and the remaining subject revealed no difference in expressed attitudes before and after. The normal approximation to the Wilcoxon test statistic indicated a z value = 2.53 which indicated that there had overall been a statistically significant effect of the talk on this measure ($p < 0.02$).

Imagine you wish to examine the responses to ordinal scale items such as the following:

What is your age group?	
Under 35	1
35–45 years	2
46–55 years	3
Over 55 years	4

by other, nominal scale, variables which represent three or more categories, such as the following:

Q4	Where is your practice located?
Inner city	1
Suburban area	2
Rural area	3

One possible analysis would be a cross-tabulation. However, this would involve a table with 4 × 3 cells, that is, 12 cells, and you are likely to run into the problem of small cell expected frequencies. Where ordinal variables are involved and the grouping variable consists of three or more categories as is shown above (Q4), the Kruskal–Wallis test may be used. This is an equivalent of the one way analysis of variance procedure for ordinal scale items and will indicate whether doctors at the three types of practice have responded differently. This analysis is suitable for testing for between-group differences when the samples do not come from normal populations, or when the population variances are widely different (heterogeneous), and is also suitable for data arising from ordinal scales. The Kruskal–Wallis H statistic is approximated by the chi-squared distribution. If a number of measurements has the same value, these are called tied ranks and a correction factor needs to be calculated, which is applied

The Kruskal–Wallis test

A clinical psychology student carried out a trial using three groups. All were out-patient service users diagnosed with mild to moderate anxiety. One group was assigned as a control group and was not given active treatment; a second group was given a series of cognitive-behavioural therapy (CBT) sessions and a third group was given biofeedback (BFT) sessions. All clients were randomised to one of these three groups. The principal outcome measure was the score on a 10 point ordinal scale measuring subjective anxiety levels at the end of the course of treatment. There were limited facilities for the cognitive-behavioural interventions and only six patients were able to be treated with this intervention. The following data was obtained.

Control	CBT	BFT
7	5	3
6	8	4
6	4	3
4	3	2
8	4	4
5	3	5
9		7
5		4
6	4	4 *Median*

An examination of the median anxiety scores from the clients in this pilot study indicated to the psychologist that both forms of active intervention appeared promising and were worth further investigation. The Kruskal–Wallis test indicated that, overall, there were statistically significant group differences (chi-square = 6.96, DF = 2, $P < 0.05$).

automatically by some statistical analysis packages in the case of tied ranks. However, if there are very many tied ranks, as can occur using an ordinal scale, care should be taken in interpreting this analysis if the significance is borderline. An example of data analysed using this test is indicated next.

Analysing data from interval and ratio scales

Other items in questionnaires may be measured at the ratio level, for example, answers to the following questions:

| Q5 | What is your height, please? | _____ metres |
| Q6 | What is your weight, please? | _____ kilograms |

Assuming the data is not highly skewed in nature for these items, that is, there is a reasonably equal spread around the mean, with most people providing values near the mean, parametric tests of significance of differences between means may be appropriate. If you wish to compare the means of this type of data between two groups, for example males and females in the sample, the independent groups *t* test may be used. If there are three or more groups, and you wish to determine overall whether the mean values of the groups significantly differ, the one way ANOVA (analysis of variance) procedure is appropriate. The one way ANOVA will provide an *F* value which will indicate, overall, whether the means of the various groups are significantly different. Other examples of the application of the *t* test and the one way ANOVA are shown next.

Experimental data also frequently involves the collection of interval or ratio scale information, such as the determination of blood glucose or cholesterol levels, or the measurements of aerobic capacity. If it is a simple two independent groups design, the independent groups *t* test may be employed. If the experiment involves making two measurements on the same individuals under different conditions of the independent variable, the data is 'paired' and the appropriate analysis is the paired *t* test. Examples of each are indicated next.

The two independent groups t test

Sixteen subjects were recruited to an experiment where the effects of controlled periods of daily exercise on a measure of aerobic capacity (VO_{2max}) were determined. The subjects were matched pairwise on initial aerobic capacity and subsequently one of each pair was randomly allocated to an experimental or a control group. This ensured that the groups were comparable initially. Eight subjects were therefore allocated to a control group and eight to the experimental (exercising) group. One subject dropped out of the experimental group leaving the following measurements which were recorded. The data which was analysed represents the VO_{2max} determinations in each group at the end of the experiment as follows:

Experimental Group	Control Group
20.3	18.2
21.3	15.4
34.6	15.3
18.4	17.3
16.5	14.1

22.8	19.8
21.7	20.2
	18.5

The mean of the experimental group was therefore 22.23 units and the mean of the control group was 17.35 units. The equal variance two group t test was used which indicated that these two means were just significantly different ($t = 2.19$, DF= 13, $P < 0.05$).

The paired t test

Twelve volunteers were assessed on their psychomotor ability. The independent variable being investigated was the effect of practice on the task. Measurements were therefore taken on the number of performance errors on the task prior to the start of the experiment and at the end of the experiment as follows:

Subject	Errors before	Errors after
1	6	5
2	4	2
3	3	4
4	6	5
5	2	2
6	6	3
7	4	1
8	3	3
9	2	1
10	5	4
11	5	5
12	3	2

The mean number of errors before the practice was therefore 4.08 and this dropped to 3.08 following the training. A paired t test indicated that this difference was statistically significant ($t = 2.87$, DF= 11, $P < 0.02$), indicating an effect of the practice. The correlation between the two sets of measurements was $r = 0.68$ ($P < 0.02$), indicating that subjects who tended to perform relatively well the first time round also did relatively well on the second measurement and those who tended to make a lot of errors on first testing also tended to do so on second testing.

Very often, more than two experimental conditions of an independent variable are needed. For example, in an exercise fitness testing experiment using cycle ergometers, six different load conditions were used with the same group of subjects in an experiment where the dependent variable was the heart rate in beats per minute. Here, a repeated measures one way ANOVA was used for the following data.

The one way repeated measures ANOVA

Ten volunteers were screened for fitness and took part in an experiment where they pedalled on an exercise ergometer under six conditions of the independent variable (the loading). Heart rate monitors were attached and the heart rate in beats per minute was the dependent variable.

Load conditions

1.0 kg	1.5 kg	2.0 kg	2.5 kg	3.0 kg	3.5 kg
91.00	101.00	116.00	132.00	147.00	164.00
88.00	102.00	125.00	141.00	164.00	181.00
76.00	112.00	140.00	155.00	175.00	192.00
93.00	98.00	101.00	118.00	130.00	149.00
94.00	95.00	109.00	126.00	145.00	160.00
90.00	101.00	123.00	131.00	149.00	170.00
80.00	93.00	115.00	127.00	140.00	158.00
99.00	106.00	111.00	136.00	152.00	167.00
98.00	100.00	118.00	143.00	180.00	191.00
87.00	98.00	105.00	127.00	151.00	166.00

A repeated measures one way ANOVA indicated a highly significant F value = 149.6 (5,45) ($P < 0.001$). The degrees of freedom are presented as the between conditions DF(5) and the error or within conditions DF(45).

Sometimes experiments involve three or more independent groups and you wish to determine the significance of differences in mean values of the dependent variable between the groups. Assuming the assumptions of the parametric ANOVA are met, the independent groups one way ANOVA may be used as shown next.

The one way independent groups ANOVA

A psychologist was concerned to investigate the effects of distraction on the performance of a task which involved solving a wooden block puzzle. The dependent variable was the time taken in seconds to solve the puzzle and the independent variable was no distraction (condition 1), auditory distraction only (condition 2) and auditory and visual distraction (condition 3). Thirty subjects were chosen and ten were randomly allocated to each condition. The results are shown below.

No distraction	Auditory distraction	Auditory and visual distraction
16	14	16
21	23	31
15	18	28
14	28	27
19	19	22
17	24	19
11	17	33
9	12	28
26	20	27
12	16	34

The mean times taken to solve the puzzle were 16 seconds in condition 1, 19.1 seconds in condition 2 and 26.5 seconds in condition 3. The one way ANOVA indicated, overall, that these means were significantly different and the F value was 10.46 with 2 and 27 degrees of freedom ($P < 0.0005$).

The effect of two or more independent variables may need to be examined in experimental work. For example, a researcher wished to examine the effect of prior experience on the number of errors made by ward clerks during the introduction of a new computerised system of record keeping in the region. Twelve staff who had experience of the old system were selected together with twelve staff who had no experience of this. Six staff from each group were randomly selected and allocated either to use the new system or use the old system which used different software. The dependent variable was the number of data entry errors made by each group in one week. The results obtained can be seen below.

The two way independent groups ANOVA

System	Experience	Errors	Mean errors made
Old system	No	4, 5, 6, 6, 8, 5	5.67

Old system	Yes	1, 1, 2, 3, 2, 1	1.67
New system	No	5, 6, 4, 6, 5, 7	5.50
New system	Yes	10, 7, 8, 6, 7, 9	7.83

A two way factorial analysis of variance was carried out. There were no significant main effects of experience ($F(1,20) = 1.67$, $P = 0.1$) but the main effect of type of system used was significant ($F(1,20)$ $P < 0.001$) and there was a significant interaction of the two independent variables ($F(1,20) = 41.49$, $P < 0.001$). That is, the analysis is indicating that the mean errors of the experienced group were not significantly different from the mean number of errors made by the inexperienced group, when these are averaged over both the old and the new systems. The mean errors made on the new system were, however, significantly higher than the mean errors made using the old system. There was a greater number of errors made on the new system, but this was only true of the group who had been used to the old system. The experienced group made fewest errors on the old system but the greatest number of errors on the new system – this is what the significant interaction effect is indicating.

An experimental design which therefore simultaneously takes two or more independent variables, or factors, into account therefore has the advantage of enabling interactions between the variables to be determined. In this example, the health researcher concluded that the previously learned skills had been detrimental to learning the new software, perhaps because the experienced clerks had overlearned the necessary old skills and found them hard to 'unlearn'.

Many other possible designs are encountered in experimental work. Mixed models are frequent; for example, a two way mixed design would involve one independent factor and one repeated measures factor. A two way repeated measures ANOVA would involve two independent variables each having repeated measures; this design can be economical of research subjects when they are scarce. Three way and higher ANOVA models are also encountered in practice. As has been emphasised already, it is preferable in student projects to keep designs simple, as interpreting the meaning of statistically significant multiway interactions between variables can be problematical.

Referring once more to Figure 8.2, associations between variables when the data has been measured at an interval or ratio level involve the Pearson correlation coefficient for pairs of variables and multiple regression techniques when combinations of variables are involved. Pearson correlation coefficients may be calculated on this type of data, in order to determine the size and direction of the association. The Pearson value varies between 0 (no association) and +1 (both variables completely positively associated) and –1 (a perfect negative association). In the example given earlier, there is likely to be a significant positive association, or correlation, between height and weight. Correlational analysis is only appropriate, however, if the variables are linearly associated; that is, a scatterplot indicates the pairs of values are distributed more or less around a straight line which could be drawn through them, as is shown in Figure 8.10. If your particular variables indicate a non-linear association, you will need to take the advice of a statistician regarding their analysis.

Correlation analysis is only appropriate if all the observations are independent, so only one

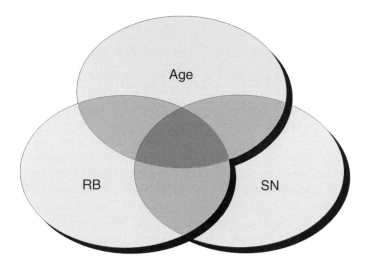

Figure 8.3   Venn diagram illustrating a partial correlation. When the effects of age (dark shaded area) are removed, the strength of the correlation between religious belief (RB) and social networking (SN) is reduced.

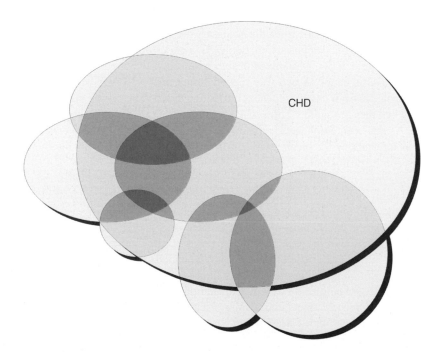

Figure 8.4   Venn diagram illustrating the interaction of six independent variables (small ellipses)on CHD rates.

measurement on each variable should come from one individual. It is important to appreciate that a statistically significant correlation implies no causal link between the variables but simply that high values of one are associated with high (or low) values of the other variable. There may be another confounding variable, which may not even have been measured, which may be 'causing' the two variables under consideration to vary together, as are illustrated in Figure 3.2. Another misuse of correlation analysis occurs when 'fishing expeditions' are carried out on the data. That is, there may be measurements of many variables which have been made and it is not uncommon to correlate each variable with all the others in large correlation matrices and to pick out the few which may be statistically significant. There may be no hypothesis or explanation for why they are related and the chances are that some spurious correlations will emerge in these circumstances.

Multiple associations between variables

Correlation analysis is a bivariate technique, that is, the relationship between pairs of variables is being explored. When the relationship between a dependent or outcome variable is being explored in relation to two or more independent variables, we are in the area of multivariate analysis. A frequently employed technique here is multiple regression and this technique is briefly considered below. Another possibility is partial correlation analysis. This allows the investigator to examine the relationship between pairs of variables, whilst holding the effects of other variables constant. The technique is very useful, therefore, to identify potential confounding variables. For example, age is often a confounding variable in studies. For example, if a straightforward bivariate (also known as zero-order) correlation were to be discovered in a survey between strength of religious belief and the amount of social networking people engaged in, we could hypothesise that people who were generally older tended both to have greater religious belief and also more social networks. That is, the relationship could be partly spurious and a partial correlation analysis could be carried out removing (or 'controlling for') the effects of age by taking all three variables into account in the analysis. This effect is shown diagrammatically in Figure 8.3.

Another commonly used multivariate technique is multiple regression analysis which is used to determine the relative contribution of several independent variables to the dependent. One of the principal reasons for conducting this analysis is to ask how well the independent variables explain the dependent. For example, an association between coronary heart disease mortality and the number of cigarettes smoked could be explored by bivariate correlation and a Pearson r value calculated. A simple (independent–dependent) regression analysis could also be conducted to calculate r^2 which indicates how well a best fitting straight line through the points represents the relationship of the two variables. In practice, there are many other factors that impinge upon CHD mortality rates, such as obesity, dietary saturated fat intake, genetic predisposition and so forth. Assuming the data was available on each of these independent variables, a multiple regression analysis could be conducted. In analogous fashion to the calculation of r^2 with two variables, multiple regression enables the calculation of a multiple coefficient known as R^2 which indicates how well all of the independent variables in combination explain the values of the dependent.

The Venn diagram in Figure 8.4 illustrates the concept pictorially. Here the variance in the dependent variable, CHD rates, illustrated by the large ellipse, is partly explained by the various independent variables such as number of cigarettes smoked, grammes of dietary fat intake and so on. Some of these independent variables are correlated with each other (and hence overlap in the diagram), although the independent variables should not exhibit very high correlations in a regression analysis. Some independent variables, or predictors in a regression equation, will explain a greater proportion of the variance in the dependent than others, illustrated in Figure 8.4 by the varying sizes of the ellipses. Not all of the variance in the dependent variable is ever explained by the combined effect of the independents (the larger the R^2 value the greater this is) as there are always other factors involved, not all of which may have been measured or even be recognised at present.

Multiple regression analysis is not a straightforward technique and if you have a data analysis problem which indicates its potential application, as outlined above, you are advised to consult a statistical adviser regarding its use and interpretation.

Deciding on an analysis

When considering the analysis of your data, you should thus be clear about the answers to a number of questions, including those that follow.

● What is the level of measurement employed: nominal, ordinal, interval or ratio?
● If interval or ratio scales have been employed, does the data come from a population which is approximately normally distributed?
● How many groups are there: one, two or more than two?
● Are the data repeated measures, e.g. before and after measurements on the same individuals?
● Do you wish to *describe* data, examine *differences* between groups, *associations* between variables or provide an answer to another question?

The level of measurement, as has been emphasised above, will help determine which statistical procedures may be applied, mainly by limiting the possibilities if the scales employed were not interval or ratio, which is frequently the case, for example, in questionnaire instruments. If the measurements are highly skewed, based upon initial exploration of the data, you are advised to stay clear of many parametric procedures such as the analysis of variance. Whether a particular analysis such as the *t* test or the one way analysis of variance is appropriate will frequently depend upon the number of groups involved. As has been indicated, there are alternative forms of each of these tests which are appropriate if the data represents independent groups or repeated measures on the same group of individuals. Within these constraints, there may be choices of alternative analyses which will depend upon the aims of the study and the questions you wish to address in the analysis.

Some other considerations

Samples are normally drawn from a particular population, with characteristics of interest to the study in question. In order to determine whether the mean of one group is significantly different from the mean of another, as has been discussed, a test of significance of differences between means is needed in order to assess whether any variations in the means can reasonably be attributed to chance (the 'null hypothesis') or whether they represent a real ('statistically significant') difference. Two-tailed tests of significance are normally chosen, that is, the assumption is made that the difference could occur in either direction. The widely used *t* test for interval or ratio scale measurements assumes that the samples are random samples from normal (or approximately normal) distributions and, further, the equal variance t test assumes that the populations have equal variances. This is a parametric test and, unless its assumptions can be met, it is safer to use a non-parametric equivalent (either the Mann–Whitney test for independent groups or the Wilcoxon test if the data is paired).

Association of variables can be explored with Pearson correlations for two variables and multiple linear regression is appropriate where there may be several independent variables and one dependent variable. More advanced techniques may also be appropriate. There is a regression analysis called logistic regression which is appropriate when the dependent variable is a binary variable such as disease present or absent. Item analysis of questionnaires may employ factor analytic techniques such as principal components analysis, which is a data reduction technique that aims to identify clusters of factors from a large number of items. These analyses are beyond the scope of the introductory statistics discussed here and advice should be sought from a statistician if you think you may need to employ them.

Non-parametric tests are appropriate where the data comes from a population with a highly skewed, that is, non-normal, distribution. We can make use of exploratory data analysis procedures to help determine which type of subsequent analysis is appropriate. These procedures include the production of box plots and normality plots of data and goodness-of-fit tests, such as the Kolmogorov–Smirnov test, on data in order to determine numerically whether there is a significant departure from normality.

The results of these normality tests should be interpreted along with other information about the distribution of the variables. Thus, when the sample size is large, any goodness-of-fit test is likely to lead to a rejection of the null hypothesis, that is, it will indicate rejection of normality, simply because of the existence of a large number of accumulated small departures from normality, even when the data may be suitable for parametric analyses. A visual examination of the distribution of a variable by means of a histogram is often informative, and many packages enable the facility to superimpose a normal curve on the histogram, as is shown in Figure 7.3.

It needs to be borne in mind that there may be other assumptions for particular analyses which need to be met, apart from assumptions about the distribution of the data. Multiple regression analysis, for example, may not be meaningful if there exists a high degree of intercorrelation (multicollinearity) between the various independent variables, and analysis of variance procedures makes assumptions about the equivalence (homogeneity) of the variances of the variables involved. Data gathered in practice is rarely perfect in meeting all the assumptions of tests but you should be aware of what these are. The degree to which these assumptions may be stretched depends in part upon the robustness of the tests used and tests such as the t test are generally regarded as having a high degree of robustness.

Confidence intervals

One topic in statistics which has not been introduced yet is the idea of confidence intervals. Measurements are carried out on samples which are drawn from the larger population of interest. The population may be defined as any group sharing some characteristic, such as patients with certain diagnostic signs, people aged over 65 and so on. In a laboratory study, the population may be the totality of machine events at particular settings, from which a particular sample of measurements will be drawn. The mean value observed in a sample is our best estimate of the real value in the population, but if a different sample had been drawn a slightly different mean value may have been obtained. The extent to which the sample mean will accurately reflect the population mean will depend upon the size of the sample; larger samples will reduce chance statistical fluctuations or random error. Bias, or systematic error, may also be present in a sample which is not representative of the population. Assuming repeated random (that is, unbiased) samples were to be drawn from the population, it can be shown that the distribution of the mean values of the samples would be approximately normal. The standard error of the mean (SEM) provides an indication of the variability amongst many possible sample means. This characteristic enables us to make an estimate of the uncertainty associated with a single sample estimate of the true population value. This measure of uncertainty is known as a confidence interval and represents the range of values within which we can be confident, at a particular degree of probability, that the true population value lies. A 95 per cent confidence interval is frequently quoted.

Confidence intervals are applied to many different types of sample estimates including proportions, and can be invaluable in assisting the interpretation of the data. Many journals stipulate that confidence intervals associated with effect sizes are presented along with data, where appropriate. The importance of this is emphasised by Gore and Altman:

> Careful reporting does not end at significance testing, especially when the author's summary is that the difference between treatments is not statistically significant (p > 0.05). What that amounts to is a statement that the trial results are consistent with there being no difference between treatments, and is not at all the same as saying that there is actually no difference. The distinction becomes clear if the authors report also the range from the smallest to the largest effect of treatment with which the trial data are consistent – a 95 per cent confidence interval for example. This range includes zero when the difference between treatments is not statistically significant ($p > 0.05$) but accommodates also real positive and negative differences. If we assumed that the actual treatment effect is outside the 95 per cent limits and were to test the data from that viewpoint, we would conclude that the outcome of the trial was improbable.... This is often a highly informative conclusion but is suppressed by mere testing of significance.
>
> (Gore and Altman 1982:73)

Some words of caution

From everything that has been said, it should be clear that erroneous and misleading results can be reported by the incorrect application of statistical procedures. Sometimes this may arise from incomplete understanding of the necessary processes involved and I have been concerned to emphasise that expert statistical help should be sought whenever there is any doubt about the correct procedures. However, there are some fundamental rules that all quantitative researchers should be aware of. In particular, it is a common enough mistake to collect data and then subject it to extensive analyses 'to see what emerges'. This type of data trawling exercise is fraught with statistical pitfalls. Conducting repeated analyses is likely to generate some 'false positive' conclusions, that is, the possibility of a Type I error is increased. It is not uncommon, for example, to correlate many variables together and then explain, on the basis of statistical significance, the hypothesised basis of the relationships. We expect on average about 5 per cent of tests conducted to be statistically significant at the 5 per cent level. To trawl the data in this way, and only to report statistically significant findings, is a dishonest approach.

A much better approach is to decide in advance what analyses are appropriate and to

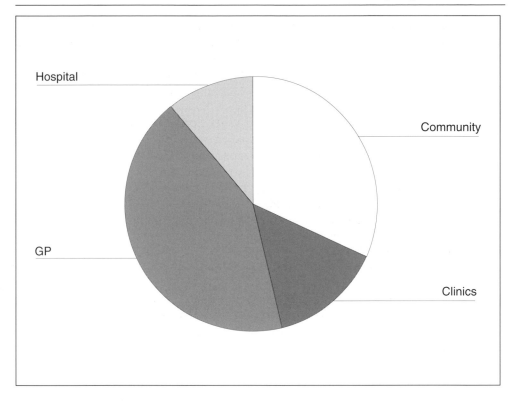

Figure 8.5 Pie chart indicating the percentage of patients seen in community, clinic, general practice and hospital settings.

conduct the analysis with certain questions in mind. In experimental studies, this will be based upon the hypotheses being tested, but the same approach is appropriate for the analysis and reporting of survey data, for instance. There is a place for additional exploratory analyses in order to point to directions for further systematic investigation but these *post hoc* analyses should not be reported as definitive evidence.

A related problem concerns results of studies which are actually published; it is recognised that there exists a reporting bias, or publication bias, in that only 'positive' or 'statistically significant' studies tend to get reported. It should be emphasised, however, that studies which show no statistically significant differences are likely to be just as important and the reasons why no differences were evident can deserve careful discussion. These studies should not be regarded as 'failures' but can be reported with equal confidence, assuming steps have been taken to minimise biases in the usual way.

Presenting the results

Most statistical analysis packages calculate an exact probability value associated with the computation of a test statistic. This probability value is expressed in the following way: for example, $P = 0.031$ or $P = 0.086$. If $P < 0.05$, we can reject chance as a reasonable explanation for the results and accept the alternative or research hypothesis. A probability of $P = 0.05$ is indicating that there is a 5 per cent chance that the results could have occurred by chance;

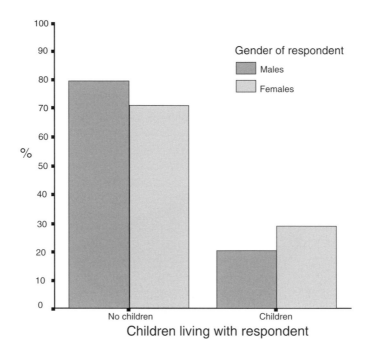

Figure 8.6 Clustered bar chart indicating the percentage of male and female survey respondents who each had children living with them.

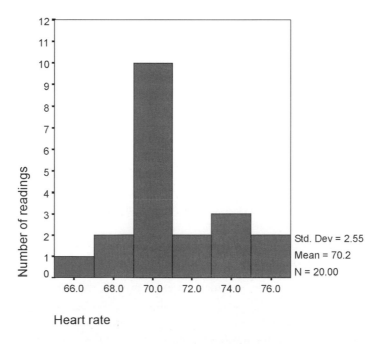

Figure 8.7 Histogram representing twenty consecutive readings of heart rate in one subject.

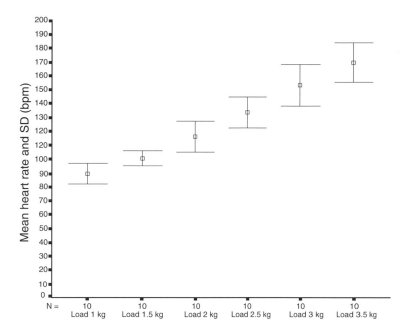

Figure 8.8 Error bar chart indicating the means and standard deviations of heart rates of subjects using cycle ergometers under increasing load conditions.

another way to look at this is to say that, if the experiment were to be repeated twenty times, we could expect these results purely by chance on one occasion. Most statistics packages quote an exact probability value associated with the computation of a test statistic such as $P = 0.009$. This value should not normally be quoted in your report, however, but you should observe the convention adhered to in the scientific literature that probability values are quoted as *less than* the nearest preferred value, usually ending in 1, 2, 25 or 5. The computer output of $P = 0.009$ should therefore become $P < 0.01$ in your report. One reason that packages provide an exact P value is that sometimes it can be appropriate to quote this in a report. This may be the case if significance is almost reached, where you may wish to quote, say, $P < 0.06$ in your report rather than say that the results of the analysis were not significant, in order to highlight a strong trend in the data towards statistical significance. Trends in the data, if they are 'robust trends', which may be the case if statistical significance is almost reached or if there is a clear discernable pattern to the data, may be worth discussing in the project report despite the fact that statistical significance at the 5 per cent level is not reached. A strong trend in the data may be assumed if the probability level associated with the value of a test statistic is between $P = 0.05$ and $P = 0.1$. It is still unlikely that these results were the result of chance.

In the presentation of data, it is not always advisable to accept the defaults that a statistical package will produce as its output. Some packages, for example, will automatically scale the vertical axis on a chart between certain minimum and maximum values, not necessarily starting the scale at zero. In the charts produced in your report, you should normally set a minimum value of zero on the *y* axis, otherwise the size of differences between groups will be visually exaggerated if you only reproduce part of the range, as is illustrated in Chapter 7.

You should be cautious about reporting results to a higher degree of precision than is warranted by the methods used. Thus a laboratory machine may produce output perhaps to three

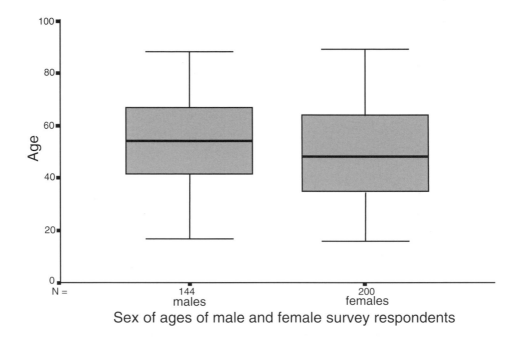

Sex of ages of male and female survey respondents

Figure 8.9   Boxplot of ages of male and female survey respondents. The dark horizontal lines indicate the median ages of males and females. The edges of the box represent the 25th and 75th percentiles and the variability outside that range is illustrated by the length of the 'whiskers'.

or four decimal places of precision, but the whole experimental procedure may be subject to an overall error of 5 per cent which is several orders of magnitude greater. To produce tables in your final report quoting values which appear to have been measured accurately down to 0.001% is therefore dishonest and misleading.

Data can be presented in the form of tables, charts or other diagrams. It is a common mistake for students to present a large number of charts displaying relatively little information on each when they could more readily be summarised as a table, which can generally present more information than a single chart. Thus a series of pie charts, which commonly display the values of single variables broken down into percentages, such as the percentages of each age group or gender who responded to a survey, could often be summarised more succinctly as a table of percentages with several columns representing the variables of interest. On the other hand, large tables can present a surfeit of information which can be difficult to grasp on first reading.

A pie chart is frequently used to display the proportion, usually as percentage, taken up by various sub-groups or categories. That is, a pie chart presents frequency data for a single variable, broken down into categories. In Figure 8.5, data from frequencies with which patients were seen in various settings, is illustrated as a pie chart.

A bar chart can be used as an alternative to a pie chart to display, by means of the heights of the bars, the numbers or percentages of people who fall into each category. A clustered bar chart enables two variables to be simultaneously displayed, that is, the values of one variable, such as whether there were children living with the survey respondents, presented separately

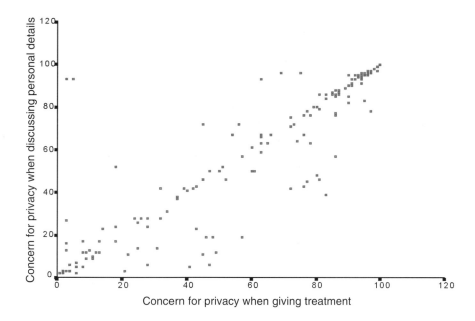

Figure 8.10 Scatterplot showing the relationship between scores obtained on two analogue rating scale questionnaire items. A correlation analysis indicated the two variables to be highly significantly associated.

by another variable such as gender. These charts can be helpful to display the results of a cross-tabulation analysis.

Do not confuse a bar chart as indicated in Figure 8.6 with a histogram as shown in Figure 8.7. A bar chart represents frequency data from categorical, that is, nominal scale variables, such as the gender dimension indicated in Figure 8.6. The horizontal, that is, x axis on a histogram represents a continuous interval or ratio scale variable. In Figure 8.7, this axis represents heart rate in beats per minute and the figures printed under each bar represent the mid-point of a range extending in either direction around this. A histogram therefore represents grouped frequency data for variables measured at interval or ratio levels of measurement. An alternative to a histogram is a frequency polygon which is a line graph representing the frequency of each value of the x axis variable.

Error bars are commonly used to display means and standard deviations or standard errors on charts. An example of an error bar chart is shown in Figure 8.7. The means of heart rates in beats per minute are indicated together with the variability extending one standard deviation on either side of the means in Figure 8.8. It can be appreciated that there is a generally increasing amount of variability associated with the higher means.

A boxplot, also known as a box-and-whisker plot, is another way of displaying a measure of central tendency – in this case the median – and the associated variability and is frequently initially used to examine the distribution of variables as an exploratory data analysis technique. An example of a boxplot is shown in Figure 8.9 which illustrates the ages associated with a sample of men and women from a questionnaire survey. The median or fiftieth percentile is indicated by the dark horizontal black bar through the boxes and the boxes represent the values falling between the twenty-fifth and seventy-fifth percentiles. Values outside that range are illustrated by the 'whiskers' extending from the boxes, so that if one whisker is longer than the other, this indicates a skew in the data in the direction of the longer whisker. The data indicates the median age of the men in the sample to be higher than that of the women.

Another way of indicating information about the variability of the data is a scatterplot, although if there is a great deal of data this can become crowded and confusing. A line graph, sometimes called an X–Y plot, plots the values of one continuous variable by another. If the points are not joined up, a scattergram is produced which plots all the individual pairs of values, as is shown in Figure 8.10. This example of a scatterplot displays a strong positive linear relationship between the two variables, and the results of the Pearson correlation analysis indicate that this association is highly significant ($r = 0.89$, $P<0.001$). Visual examination of the scatterplot, which represents the relationship between two ratio scale analogue rating scale questionnaire items on a patient satisfaction questionnaire, indicates that the two variables are linearly associated; that is, a best description of the relationship between the variables would be represented by a straight line drawn through the area of greatest clustering of the points.

Only reproduce a scatterplot with a straight line through the points if this is justified; if the relationship between the two variables is very weak the line can be misleading and can look more like an act of faith.

All charts produced should have a figure number in your report and should include an informative legend. A word about chart 'enhancements' is in order here. Most presentation graphics and statistics packages provide options to present charts with 3D and other effects. These should be avoided in scientific reports for the good reason that they generally make the chart more difficult to interpret. It is much more difficult, for example, accurately to judge the relative sizes of the slices in a three-dimensional elliptical pie chart than a straightforward one. All summary data presented in the form of tables in your report should have a table number and an informative caption. If abbreviations are used in the table, they should be explained in the caption and the significance of any differences being presented should be indicated. A table which presents data should stand alone and it can be annoying to the reader if it needs to be interpreted by referring back and forth to the main body of the text.

Action points

- Code and enter the data onto a computer.
- Work with your supervisor to discuss details of analysis.
- Conduct the analysis.
- Decide how best to present the findings in tables and charts as appropriate.

Chapter 9

Do you, Mr Jones, …?

Different types of interview

Interviews are carried out in many different guises. Thus face-to-face interviews can range from the completely unstructured to the highly structured. The entirely unstructured and non-directive interview implies that the interviewer does not shape the direction of the discussion in any way, although she may exert a facilitating influence on the discussion, for example by asking the respondent to amplify and exemplify points that are raised. This type of interaction is frequently conducted by therapists and may also be employed in research as part of the case study approach. In this approach, interviewees do not have to answer pre-set questions which may be constraining, and the data generated is thus said to be 'rich' in ethnographic terms.

On the other hand, completely unstructured, non-directed interviews can meander over the same ground back and forth and may not cover material of central interest to the research purposes. In health-related research, therefore, it is normal to have some degree of structuring to the interview. One level of structuring is known as the guided interview. The guided interviewer does not ask questions from a set list in the same order each time, but has an outline of topics to be covered and questions to be asked. The interviewer plays it by ear and decides how to work in and phrase specific questions according to the flow of the conversation. The ensuing data analysis is therefore generally easier than with completely unstructured interviews and a more or less consistent agenda is covered whilst the interviewer retains flexibility in the approach and phrasing. On the other hand, the guided interview has a number of potential disadvantages. There is room for a substantial influence of the interviewer to be imposed, consciously or unconsciously, on the outcome. This arises because the wording of questions is not standardised and there may be varying emphases from interview to interview in the way that information is obtained and questions asked, and in the interpersonal interactions.

In recognition of these influences, the semi-structured interview therefore uses a more standardised procedure. A number of psychological and psychiatric assessment procedures utilise this method, but it can be applied more generally. Initially, each person interviewed will be asked basically the same set of questions, which are drawn up in the form of a printed schedule, but there may be 'cut off' questions such that if it is inappropriate to pursue a line of enquiry, some questions may not be asked. Interviewers may also ask supplementary questions in order to assist with the interpretation of an answer, and these supplementary questions are not necessarily the same for each interviewee. Research subjects may be allowed to answer questions in an entirely 'open-ended' manner using whatever words and phrases come

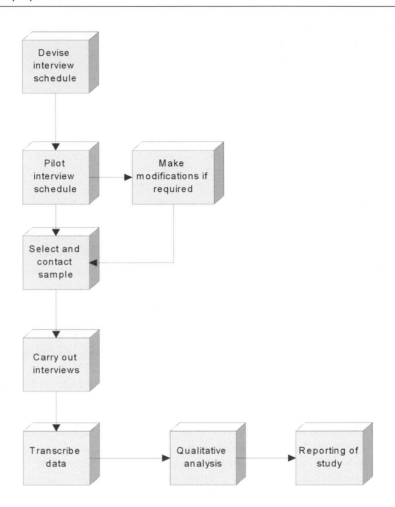

Figure 9.1   Stages involved in conducting a typical interview study.

to them, or sometimes they may be prompted in the semi-structured interview to choose between a number of standardised options. This type of interview provides data which may be of a quantitative as well as a qualitative type: all topics of interest are covered, and there is generally less room for interpersonal bias on the part of the interviewer. However, the interviewer loses some flexibility and this type of interview can appear strained and formal and far away from a conversational approach.

Finally, there is the fully structured interview. As with the semi-structured interview the wording and the order of questions are fixed. However, the respondent may only answer according to predefined scales. For example, the respondent will have been informed at the start that the answers should be provided according to the following system: Strongly agree, Agree, Unsure, Disagree or Strongly disagree or perhaps 'Always', 'Sometimes' 'Rarely' or 'Never'. If respondents talk about something else, or give reasons for their answers, this may not even be recorded by the interviewer. This type of fully structured interview essentially consists of the face-to-face administration of a closed questionnaire and as such has few, if any, advantages over using the postal system for this purpose. It is, however, frequently employed by market researchers who wish to ensure that questionnaires are filled in on the spot, either on the street or perhaps by calling at households.

The form of an interview

In any interview, apart perhaps from the completely structured kind, the quality and manner of the interviewer's interaction with the research subject plays a vital part in the conversation, and thus in the outcome of the interview and the study. It should be an aim that rapport is established early on; rapport can be influenced by such factors as the type of clothes the interviewer is wearing (which can be chosen), the age, gender and ethnicity of the interviewer (which cannot), as well as the manner and conversational style of the researcher (which can be learned). Interviewees are likely to be most comfortable using their normal language. Thus, if a researcher is conducting a set of interviews with young people concerning their street drug use, it would not be appropriate to use terms like amphetamines or benzodiazepines when street terms like 'speed' or 'downers' would be their normal language.

Remember that an interview provides an opportunity to observe and record non-verbal as well as verbal behaviour. It is relatively easy to forget, however, that the interviewer too is giving non-verbal signals which can influence the reaction to questions asked. So develop the demeanour of the disinterested 'poker player' in your interview style. You may be genuinely shocked or disgusted by something you hear from an interviewee but if this reaction is communicated to the interviewee you will significantly bias the course of the ensuing discussion. Interviews will be unlikely to be productive if subjects feel that interviewers are being judgmental about them or their answers. The purpose of any particular question can be explained in clear and straightforward terms and full information should be given at the start of the interview about the purpose and nature of the research.

In health-related investigations, the issue of confidentiality is particularly acute. In qualitative research, exemplified by the interview and case analysis approaches, it is common practice to quote some statements by research subjects verbatim in research reports. It is possible that individuals could be identified by what they have said and this may be a fear to be allayed, particularly if the research is on a sensitive issue such as sexual health or mental health. Getting subjects to 'open up' in sensitive areas may take repeated visits and a long period of establishing rapport.

The length of a research interview is an important consideration. Thus, in research proposals, it is common practice to say, for example, that ten one-hour interviews will be conducted with the client group. Like the issue of sample size discussed in Chapter 4, this figure is often plucked 'out of the air' without regard to the nature and demands of the interview on both the subject and the researcher. My advice is not to stick rigidly to a set time, because the course of an interview is usually unpredictable; it is unlikely than any research interview lasting less than 20–30 minutes is going to obtain a lot of rich, meaningful information from respondents. After all, an initial period needs to be set aside for establishing rapport in an interview situation and after 20 minutes you may barely be getting going. On the other hand, and depending upon the client group, 60–90 minutes may be as much as you can reasonably demand of the concentration, attention span and time of interviewees. Within these broad limits, there is room for flexibility depending upon the course and flow of the questions with individual research subjects.

In student work, you are often the sole interviewer. Issues of inter-rater agreement and reliability therefore may not need to be examined. However, much research involves teamwork and if more than one interviewer is to share the interviewing of the subjects, consistency and standardisation must be ensured. This could involve training in listening skills, in the way and manner of asking supplementary questions and in methods of achieving rapport. Whether you are the sole interviewer or not, however, it is highly desirable that you have some 'dry runs' before the main data collection. This could involve practising the interviews on a pilot group who may be able to provide feedback on the process. The typical steps involved in an interview study are indicated in Figure 9.1.

When it comes to asking questions, we all have some bad habits which may be difficult to rid ourselves of if they are not recognised and guarded against. Thus many people have a habit of asking a question in the following way:

'You didn't go to the doctor's last week, did you?'

when they mean:

'Did you go to the doctor's last week?'

It is easy to roll two or more questions into one.

'Was that a helpful experience or was it basically unhelpful and did you find that you wanted to go back again?'

The respondent may answer only part of a multi-part question and may find that she has forgotten the full set of questions by the time she has answered the first.

Questions like:

'Are you finding the treatment helps your angina?'

are likely to elicit little more than 'Oh, yes, definitely' or 'Not at all' in response. Open-ended questions like:

'In what ways does the treatment tackle your angina?'

will be more likely to produce a detailed and informative response. Repeating salient words of an answer which has been given, as well as non-verbal gestures such as nods and hand motions, can all be helpful in getting subjects to elaborate on answers. Listening skills are vital in a dynamic research interview. The interviewer can pick up particular unusual or meaningful words used in an answer by a respondent, as well as intonation and tone of voice, and use them to frame supplementary questions. The importance of silent pauses in a conversation may be recognised; people often feel embarrassed if a conversation leads to an extended silence but the temptation to 'fill the silence' by saying something is not always a good idea in a research interview. A research interview should be an interactive process, otherwise the strength of the method is lost. Interpretation of respondents' answers on the spot, perhaps by rephrasing their answers in your own terms and looking for a reaction, is one way of ensuring this interaction.

The importance of conducting pilot interviews cannot be over-stressed. You will probably find that your first few attempts could be considerably improved with hindsight, and opportunities to pursue and follow up interesting remarks may be lost. If you record your interviews, use a tape recorder with a separate microphone if possible and do not use a voice-activated machine. Most miniature recorders with built-in microphones pick up a lot of machine noise which can make it a difficult and tedious task to make out what was said when you come to transcribe the interviews. If you use voice activation, the recorder may not be switched on by soft-spoken interviewees, and in any case you will lose the opportunity to note the extent of any pauses in the conversation, which can be an important part of the analysis.

One of the secrets to being a good interviewer is to listen, listen and listen! Do not use the interview situation as an opportunity to argue your point of view; a research interviewer adopts a very different style from the adversarial television political interview, for example, where the aim is to put the interviewee on the spot. Listen, respond to what you hear and phrase your questions neutrally and sensitively – even if you are 'poles apart' from the views of the respondent. The aim of the research is to explain and understand the views and attitudes of the interviewees and this requires an approachable and non-confrontational attitude on the part of the researcher, whatever the issue being investigated.

Telephone interviews

Interviews can also be conducted over the telephone, giving some of the advantages of the face-to-face interview, such as the ability to follow up and explore issues raised by interviewees. However, it is generally easier for potential respondents to refuse to take part in a telephone interview than refuse face to face. Another potential, and real, disadvantage is that respondents may be reluctant to disclose personal or sensitive information over the telephone when they cannot check to whom they are speaking. Finally, of course, not everybody has a telephone at home and a sample limited to telephone subscribers is going to be particularly biased against disadvantaged low income groups, such as students. If telephone interviews are contemplated in a serious research study, it is strongly advised that postal contact explaining the purposes of the study is made with potential interviewees in advance; a call 'out of the blue' stands a fair chance of failure. In general terms, telephone interviews can be regarded as a substitute for face-to-face contact that can be justified in some circumstances, such as the collection of routine information from a client group. For example, one of my postgraduate students used the telephone interview method to collect routine follow-up data from participants on an exercise prescription scheme on a monthly basis, thus saving the time and cost involved with personal visits.

As can be appreciated from what has been said in this section, conducting a research interview is not a trivial task. To conduct successful interviews requires tact, patience and empathy together with a high level of interpersonal skills. However, many of the necessary techniques can be learned through practice and experience. Once your interviews are completed, you are left with the task of analysis and interpretation. How this may be approached is discussed in the next chapter.

Action points

- Decide on the most appropriate type of interview to conduct for your study.
- Make decisions about the numbers and type of people to interview and whether this should include professionals as well as clients or patients.

- Practise your interview technique on a pilot group who can give you feedback.
- Keep in mind the purpose of the study in designing your qualitative research and aim to collect data with the subsequent focus of the analysis in mind.

Chapter 10

Qualitative studies

If your project is primarily qualitative in nature, such as the examination of records, focus group discussions or interview transcripts, a recognised qualitative technique of data collection and analysis will be needed. This can be approached in many different ways. Qualitative projects are frequently small, detailed accounts of a few cases or a closely related situation, although projects may be longitudinal or comparative. Generally, qualitative analyses are much more time consuming to conduct than statistical analyses and are frequently less than straightforward in concept. As with quantitative procedures, you will need to justify the approach and the method of analysis adopted in your final report. Qualitative analyses can either be approached manually, which is the traditional approach, or they may be computer-assisted. In either case, it is vital that you are clear about what you are attempting to do. Qualitative methods may take a number of approaches so that, whilst some projects are clearly defined from the start, others take form and substance as data accumulates and become subject to ongoing analysis. However, all projects benefit from advance planning, although qualitative analysis is very often a process of the exploration of emerging ideas and concepts.

What is qualitative inquiry?

There are many approaches to qualitative inquiry which can range from a 'scientific' search for lawful relationships to an exploration of the 'essence' of phenomena, as in phenomenology. The over-riding characteristic of qualitative approaches, from whatever theoretical orientation, is an emphasis on the naturalness of a situation; that is, the actions, beliefs, values and meaning of real-life people and situations, in contrast to the 'artificial' controlled situation of experimental laboratories. Unlike experimental approaches, which generally adopt a reductionist strategy, qualitative approaches are 'organic' or holistic in that they attempt to integrate many features and determinants of situations and explain the interplay of people in groups, societies and organisations. Understanding meaning in these situations is essentially down to the researcher gaining a deep and empathetic grasp of what people say and how they act through direct personal observation.

It is not attempted here to discuss in depth the theoretical philosophical assumptions of the many different approaches that can be subsumed under the umbrella of qualitative inquiry. Taxonomies of qualitative appoaches have been produced around either the methods employed or the theoretical orientations, and in either case these taxonomies contain something like twenty or thirty different approaches and methods. At the risk of being simplistic, a brief overview of some influential approaches and methods is provided here. A more detailed discussion on qualitative approaches is provided in standard texts on qualitative analysis such as Miles and Huberman (1994) and Strauss and Corbin (1990).

Phenomenology aims to study the phenomena or manifestations of human experience without consideration of the contexts either of 'objective' reality or 'subjective' connotations. The phenomenological approach is contrasted with much of traditional scientific inquiry in the form of positivism. Neither speculative thinking nor the unobservable are within its remit. However, 'ideal' objects and conscious life can be made evident and thus known. Phenomenology is an approach which therefore centres on the value of individual experience in the deep practical understanding of observable matters; this is in contrast to a 'positivistic' view that external objective reality exists independent of any observer. The phenomenological approach therefore puts human consciousness at the centre of events and places less emphasis on causes and purposes of events. Thus phenomena appear within the realm of consciousness and should be examined in this context. An investigation of the delusions associated with a diagnosis of schizophrenia for example, from a phenomenological perspective, could concentrate upon the internal experiences of the patients in terms of their consciousness and feelings rather than pointing out 'logical' inconsistencies in the delusions.

Phenomenology is a tradition in philosophy, originating about a century ago from the writings of Edmund Husserl, aiming to study the essential aspects of phenomena without recognition of accompanying scientific or cultural paradigms. A phenomenological approach emphasises the need to liberate the researcher from presuppositions and preconceptions about the world. Whether this is entirely possible or not is a moot point, however. Phenomenology as a philosophy aims to transcend both the traditions of idealism and realism to reach the things themselves. Idealism is a philosophical tradition stemming from Plato in which the mind is held to be the fundamental reality; realism, which exists as a fundamental pillar of the positivist tradition, holds that material objects exist independent of the perceiver.

Interactionism in various flavours has had a major impact on social theory and methodological approaches. The tradition of symbolic interactionism derives from the thinking of G.H Mead and Herbert Blumer and is concerned with the dynamic activities taking place between people, rather than either the characteristics of individuals or the links between social structures and the individual. The physical environment within which people operate acquires meaning in different ways to different people, each of whom are active acting organisms within the environment and with each other. Although we are biological organisms, the existence of symbols such as language enables us to give meaning to things in the natural world. This interpretive framework makes us human and collective actions characterise human society which is dynamic. In the study of health issues, an adoption of this approach implies a rejection of both genetic determinism, whereby the most important determiner of behaviour is deemed to be the genotype, and associated 'instincts' and extreme environmentalism as it exists, for example, in naïve behaviourism.

The ethnographic approach is a methodological approach which lays emphasis on the full description of events and actions involving people; it has a long and honourable tradition in anthropology where the aim is adequately to describe a group or culture in all its minutiae, the mundane as well as the exotic, rather than to provide a conceptual framework. Inevitably, however, analytic processes are brought to bear on the choice and description of material. Structured and unstructured observational techniques and interviews can form the source material and insights are gained as the study progresses and informs subsequent observations. The grounded theory approach is a particular method which has gained wide acceptance within the qualitative community and, although sharing some characteristics with ethnography, places rather more emphasis on theory derived from data.

The fundamental assumption of the grounded theory approach is that theories flow from the data and are not separate from it. A theory must be grounded in the material then being studied – it is not a conceptual framework within which the data is 'made to fit'. The best known protagonists of this approach are Strauss and Corbin, who have written extensively on this methodological approach. The theory is derived inductively from the data, in contrast to the deductive approaches traditionally characterising scientific investigations. That is, the process of induction enables a generalisation from the particular data to a theory with wider applicability beyond the particular data studied. Unlike an experimental scientific investigation, there are no specific hypotheses stated at the start of an investigation which are subsequently tested. The analytic process associated with a grounded theory approach is rigorous and systematic and follows a number of recognised approaches. Questions are asked of the data as analysis proceeds and data is compared continuously with other data (constant comparisons) to guide analysis. Memo writing and the use of diagrams are inherent in the process. In order to ensure the theory remains 'grounded' in the data, the process of data collection and analysis are closely bound together and subsequent phases of a study are shaped by initial findings. As a result, a grounded theory researcher will not be concerned about conducting a comprehensive literature review at the start of a study; the theory will flow from the data and not from the literature background, although relevant literature will need to be uncovered and integrated into the discussion at later stages.

The grounded theory method is essentially independent of the philosophical stance of the researcher and it has been argued that both scientific and phenomenological emphases are consistent with the use of the method.

Sources of qualitative data

The major sources of data for qualitative analyses can be summarised as:

- observational data
- open-ended questionnaire data
- textual records and documentation
- interviews
- transcripts of conversations and discussions
- diary notes.

Observational data has traditionally been the method of choice for anthropological research and is regarded by anthropologists as the fundamental method for understanding another culture: the researcher lives and works amongst the people being studied for an extended period. Observational techniques, in one form or another, are also frequently used by psychologists to record the behaviour of young children in nurseries, the residents of nursing homes and so on. Observational techniques can therefore use either the method of participant observation – whereby the researcher becomes one of the group being studied – or non-participant observation where the aim is to record notes as a disinterested outsider from the group. Participant observations are less structured and suitable for qualitative techniques of analysis.

The examination of texts and documents is a frequent source of qualitative data. In our context, data may be derived from case notes, medical records or ward round minutes. One possible type of analysis involves developing your ideas and theory as you progress and illustrating your report with case study vignettes as appropriate. The method of content analysis aims to establish a set of categories which should be derived from (rather than imposed upon) the data. Qualitative analyses may appear to be a subjective approach compared to statistical analysis of numeric data, but qualitative researchers have established ways of checking the reliability and validity of what they are attempting. Thus different coders should ideally arrive at the same results, which means that definitions of the categories should be arrived at clearly and unambiguously. Content analysis can be rather a quantitative approach to a textual analysis. In much qualitative research, small numbers of texts and documents may be analysed with the aim of understanding the participants' categories themselves.

Interview data has provided the mainstay of much qualitative research. The aim is frequently to gain an authentic understanding of people's experiences and qualitative researchers find that open-ended questions are the best way of achieving this. Many students interested in health investigations have used an interview methodology as their principal research approach and this provides opportunities for recording non-verbal behaviour as well as verbal responses. As has been pointed out in Chapter 9, interviews may be unstructured or more often guided or semi-structured, so that the researcher will have an agenda to cover whilst allowing opportunities to probe and follow up replies given. Transcripts therefore provide a major source of data for qualitative analysis. Transcripts are commonly derived from interviews, but may be derived from other sources. Published studies have, for instance, used transcripts of audio tapes of counselling sessions with the aim of analysing the interactions and the types of advice given.

Conducting a content analysis

Unlike the analysis of quantitative data, as has been already implied, there are no universally agreed recognised conventions for analysing qualitative data. Thus the approach adopted may be driven as much by theoretical orientation as by the type of data which has been collected. However, the process can be made systematic, and it is this approach that I have encouraged. One possible approach, as I have indicated, is content analysis, and this has been used for many decades to analyse the content of documents and media output. In recent years, it has been applied widely in sociological and psychological studies. Documents in this sense need not be confined to written material and can include evidence in the form of videotapes, maps and photographs, for example. A typical scheme for the analysis of interview transcripts is depicted in Figure 10.1. The figure, which is an over-simplification of the procedures in practice, nevertheless indicates clearly that the process of qualitative analysis is not linear but involves much recursive exploration and refinement of interpretations of material.

A focus is initially needed for this analysis. You may have collected, say, responses to open-ended questions on a questionnaire in the area of sexual health, for example, and you have some specific investigative aims. Such questions could centre on the extent to which what people say about safe sex is reflected in their behaviour, or the nature of the relationship between knowledge and attitudes in this field. Sometimes the focus is only decided upon after reading the responses made, in the light of the comments that have been made.

The unit of analysis is an important decision that needs to be made early on. This may be anything from a single word to a line of text, a sentence or a whole paragraph. Choosing a paragraph as the unit of analysis would not be advisable in many cases, since this is likely to include too many concepts or ideas bundled together. On the other hand, a single word (a lexical analysis) provides no context for the use of the word if that is the basic unit of analysis, but

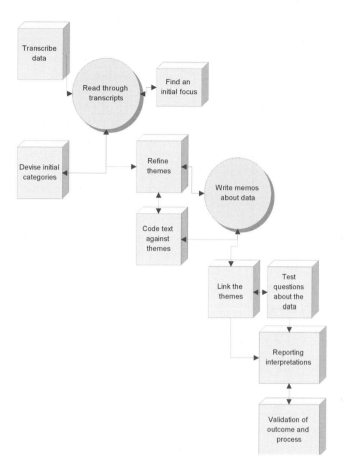

Figure 10.1 Typical stages involved in the analysis of interview transcripts.

may be important in some linguistic analyses. An alternative approach is to analyse themes in the responses, of whatever length, so long as they can be categorised in your scheme.

The content of the text may be regarded as being present at several different levels. Manifest content reflects words people actually use. On the other hand, the latent content depends upon interpretation and judgement about the content in the context in which it occurs. Inferences may be made, therefore, by the researchers about the attitudes behind certain statements, the personality characteristics of individuals and the manner in which remarks were made (e.g. tongue in cheek, jokingly, provocatively).

The decision on how to categorise the text into themes can be based upon many different schemes, such as the content or nature of the topic, the values surrounding it, the roles of the individuals participating and so on, depending upon the textual material with which one is concerned and the research purposes behind it. The category scheme is likely to evolve as the analysis proceeds. It may start off as a rough-and-ready scheme from a 'first pass' on the data and subsequently evolve so that categories become reorganised and rearranged, pruned or

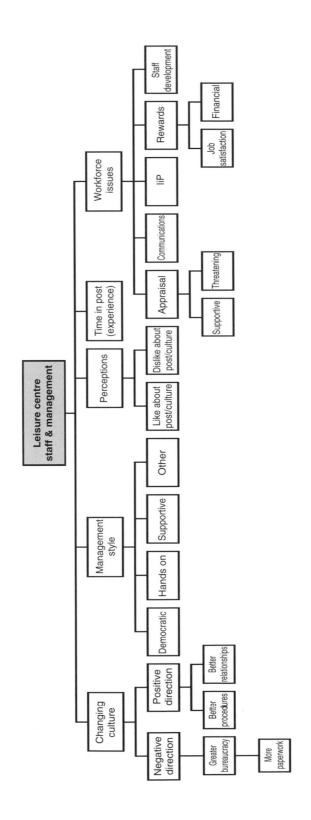

Figure 10.2 Tree diagram of categories from a content analysis.

added to as the interpretation proceeds. The process of content analysis is therefore an iterative one, and in a sense is never finished. The categories should be defined: a set of criteria for
indexing or assigning text to a particular category needs to be explicitly stated. This is important to ensure consistency of the process, and to assist reliability checking. Thus, with a dictio-
nary of definitions alongside the categories, the analysis could essentially be repeated by
another researcher. The process of conducting the content analysis centres on identifying text
units and assigning them to one or more categories as appropriate. This may be achieved manually by using different coloured highlighters on a hard copy of the transcript, or can be
assisted through the use of appropriate computer software, as is illustrated in the case study in
the following chapter. It can be a time consuming process and it is important for the remaining
stages of the analysis that is completely and thoroughly done. At the end of the coding process, a category scheme will have emerged.

An example of a category scheme representing a summary of the results of a content analysis is illustrated in Figure 10.2. This example comes from a series of interviews which were
conducted with staff at a leisure centre in the South of England with the aim of identifying
management styles in relation to the working culture of the organisation. The steps involved
in the analysis of this data, using a computerised technique, are illustrated in the next chapter.
In essence, the basic analysis was guided by the focus of the questions asked during the interviews which centred on a number of themes around the issue of the investigation which was to
examine the impact of management styles upon the culture of the organisation (a leisure
centre). Members of staff at all levels in the organisation were interviewed concerning
changes in culture, management styles, perceptions about job roles and day-to-day as well as
strategic issues concerning staff development, the Investors in People initiative and related
issues.

The category scheme depicted in Figure 10.2 is essentially hierarchically arranged in that
specific categories are subsumed under more general categories. However, these tree diagrams can depict many alternative relationships between themes, such as temporal,
aetiological or logical links. The tree diagram shown in Figure 10.2 has been shown to four
levels; more detail is certainly possible and some schemes can become very complex and
extend to many more levels. This categorisation of the raw data into 'boxes' is merely one
stage of a content analysis of this type. Further stages of analysis concentrate upon linking the
categories together, as is described below.

The purpose of a content analysis is adequately to describe and interpret textual material. The
categories which have been created should be related to each other in an appropriate manner in
order to reach conclusions about the topic under investigation. This may be achieved in a
number of distinct ways as appropriate to the data under consideration, for example:

- observing the recurrence of themes in the data
- discovering logical relationships between two or more of the categories
- developing aetiological links between the categories
- relating the findings to theory, including the generalisability of the data.

In the example illustrated in the tree diagram in Figure 10.2, the categories changing cul-
ture/negative direction/greater bureaucracy and perceptions/dislike about post or culture were
clearly related in that the same text tended to be coded under each; that is, the staff who tended
to dislike the post very often complained of the bureaucracy of the organisation. This is only

one example of the links between these categories. Thus category analysis of the data is an important part of reaching conclusions about textual material.

Content analysis can be a quantitative approach to a qualitative analysis; statistical analysis of data can occur, such as counting the frequency of occurrence of words and themes and relating these, using statistical techniques, to other variables such as gender or location of respondents. There are many other methods of analysing and presenting qualitative material other than formal content analysis. Sometimes the requirement is simply to supplement quantitative data which may have been collected, for example, using closed response questions on the same questionnaire, by augmenting the statistics with apt and appropriate extracts or quotations from the qualitative data. Some practitioners view a qualitative analysis as more of an art than a science and prefer intuitive approaches to systematic approaches.

It is probably true that much qualitative analysis remains closer to the data and to common sense than statistical analyses, which can be regarded as several steps removed from the phenomena they measure. It is important that working with qualitative data, as indeed with quantitative material, should not become a mechanical or unthinking process; the researcher is very much a close interactive partner with the data. Notes, or memos, can be written at all stages concerning ideas and concepts about the data and will eventually prove invaluable when putting together your report. The memos represent developments of your theorising as ideas come to you during the process of reading and coding the data. The memos should be kept separate from the data as they represent interpretations of the data and are therefore one or more steps removed from the material being considered. The memos can therefore be modified or discarded at later stages as the analysis unfolds.

The presentation of your qualitative analysis, like the analyses themselves, can take many different forms. The category tree display illustrated in Figure 10.2 is one method of displaying part of an analysis. As I have said, these tree diagrams can represent conceptual, temporal, aetiological, logical or many other types of relationship between the categories or, indeed, a combination of one or more of these. Other forms of qualitative data presentation include maps, diagrams, flow charts or matrices representing a classification of two sets of categories in tabular form. The reporting of much qualitative analysis, however, relies on textual description, often illustrated by appropriate and relevant quotations from the raw data.

Checking reliability and validity

As has already been indicated, there are recognised ways of checking the reliability and validity of what you are attempting in qualitative analysis. Reliability refers to the degree of consistency with which instances are assigned to the same categories by different researchers or by the same researcher on different occasions. Thus it is advisable to have the text assigned to each category checked by an independent observer to assess reliability. Reliability of observational data can also be independently assessed by comparing observations from two or more observers: this is known as inter-rater or inter-observer reliability. The reliability of interview procedures can be assisted by thorough piloting of schedules, the training of interviewers to agreed procedures and standards (if more than one interviewer will be collecting the data) and inter-rater reliability checks on the coding of answers to open-ended questions.

Validity in qualitative analysis has been defined as the extent to which an account accurately represents the particular phenomenon to which it refers. Spurious associations should be guarded against. For example, what people sometimes say in response to questions posed at an interview does not necessarily imply what they believe or how they actually behave in naturally-occurring situations. Sometimes answers are given, especially in 'formal' interview situations, which are deemed the socially acceptable response rather than reflecting the respondent's true feelings. Similarly, it has been a weakness of some qualitative work for researchers to tend to select data to fit a preconceived idea about the phenomenon under consideration, ignoring data which does not conveniently illustrate this. It is also a flaw to select field data because it is somehow 'exotic' or particularly outstanding in some way at the expense of perhaps more mundane data that is indicative of the phenomenon in question.

These general issues of validity have probably been given less detailed attention than in quantitative research, but many considerations are similar in both approaches. These include the need to be aware of:

- the impact of the research on the setting (the Hawthorne effect)
- the values and attitudes of the researcher
- the truth or otherwise of the respondent's answers.

One recognised way of checking the validity of what you are doing in qualitative research is to take your findings back to the people being studied. This is known as respondent validation and, it has been argued, is helpful in establishing confidence in the validity of the researcher's interpretation. The general concept of 'triangulation' is sometimes used by qualitative researchers to check validity. Here different methods, often drawn from different theoretical perspectives, should converge on the same, or similar, conclusions about the phenomenon being studied. For example, data from observational methods and interviews may be compared.

The ethos of much qualitative research is to regard individuals as people rather than research subjects and to conduct research *among* people rather than *on* them. The researcher is often more subjectively involved and this is reflected in the approach to the treatment and analysis of the data. Fieldwork and analysis tend to move forward in a complementary fashion and the writing proceeds as an essential part of the research process. In putting together a report adopting a qualitative method, whether to intermingle description and interpretation or keep them separate is partly a matter of personal style. In a sense, a qualitative study is never concluded and if you work towards a set of definitive conclusions you may be going beyond the limits of your material. Thus, with textual material, there is usually scope for further or different interpretations to be made, whereas with a set of numbers in a spreadsheet it is possible in principle and in practice exhaustively to analyse their relationships. In qualitative analysis, you should be especially vigilant about going beyond the evidence and making pronouncements based on personal value judgements.

It may be appreciated that qualitative analysis can be a very conceptually demanding task. It has not been possible to give you more than a flavour of some of the processes involved in this chapter. If your data is likely to need an in-depth qualitative analysis, you are advised to consult some of the references on specialised methods referred to in Chapter 18. In order to enable the reader to gain a 'feel' for some of the processes involved in a qualitative content analysis, the next chapter provides an example of a computer-assisted method of analysing interview transcripts.

Action points

- Read relevant books on your chosen method.
- Transcribe all recorded conversations using a word processor.
- Decide how best to approach your qualitative data treatment.
- Address the issues of the reliability and validity of your data.

Chapter 11

Using qualitative analysis software

Computer-assisted qualitative analyses can be accomplished with the help of specialised software. Remember that while the computer can assist you with the systematic process of thematic classification and extraction, the major conceptual tasks in qualitative analyses – theory generation and ultimately making sense of the data – are still up to you. Your data will need to be in machine-readable format, so all conversations, interview data and so on need to be accurately transcribed using a word processor as the first stage in a qualitative analysis. As a novice researcher, you should aim to allow some three to four hours for each hour of tape recorded conversation to accomplish this process.

Qualitative analysis software provides facilities to organise and manage, to explore and to search the text of documents. It can assist the process of exploring ideas about the data, linking ideas and helping to construct and test theories about the data. It will also generate reports including statistical summaries concerning the frequency of occurrences of key words and themes if necessary. Some packages, such as the WinMAX package, enable numeric variables to be set up which have been derived from the data; these variables can then be exported as files and further analysed using packages such as SPSS.

At the simplest level, therefore, specialist computer software can be an aid to the storage and retrieval of text and can consequently be used like a 'smart' filing cabinet by automating repetitive tasks such as searching through transcripts for key words. Tasks of locating and collecting together all occurrences of a key term or phrase can be accomplished and tables generated on the frequency of occurrences. You will, however, need to go further in your qualitative analysis and wish to interrogate the data and develop ideas about it. Complex or simple questions can therefore be asked about the unstructured data and concepts can be defined and linked with the material which has been gathered. You will need to decide whether the time spent learning the software is worthwhile in terms of the potential benefits. These are discussed below.

When computer programs to assist with the process of qualitative analysis first became available in the 1980s, there was a high degree of enthusiasm in some quarters about their potential. In the 1990s, qualitative data analysis software started generating differences and debate amongst the qualitative analysis community. Whilst most would agree that the software is a basic aid to assist with data management, that is, the storage and retrieval of text, opinions are divided about the usefulness and applications of programs which are designed to assist the interpretation of text. It has been stated that the software distances the researcher from the data and may constrain the methods of analysis. The majority of qualitative researchers would advocate a critical and informed approach to the software. In a similar way to the possibility of running statistical analyses on a computer without any real understanding of either the data or the methods of analysis, the idea that qualitative analysis can be automated is undermining to the task of qualitative researchers.

One set of issues revolves around the impact of the software on the research process. There is a potential threat that the questions which are asked in a qualitative project could be shaped, at least in part, by the facilities available on a particular package. There is also a suspicion in some quarters that qualitative packages tend to shift the analytic process in the quantitative direction. This suspicion arises because qualitative analysis software makes more explicit the processes through which conclusions are reached about the material under investigation. They encourage analytical rigour and visibility in the analysis, for example in the tracking of all intermediate stages leading to the final interpretations. In this way they can provide an 'audit trail' for other researchers to follow. However, it has been argued that this feature may encourage conformity rather than innovation.

Most qualitative analysis packages are based upon a grounded theory approach, whereby the conclusions and interpretations are thoroughly grounded in, or derived from, the actual material being considered, rather than from some conceptual scheme which is imposed upon it. A typical package will require all textual material to be transcribed using a word processor and then imported as a plain text file into the analysis software. At that stage, a scheme of categories or general themes may be determined, perhaps with the assistance of the word search facilities of the software. It is then typical to proceed to the stage known as 'coding' the data against the categories, that is, identifying relevant segments of text to assign to each category. Users of qualitative software have sometimes complained that it is possible to get bogged down in this process of coding, resulting in far too many coding categories, which merely leads to procrastination in conducting the actual analysis and interpretation. A well known commentator, Ian Dey (1993), has warned of the over-fragmentation possible at the coding stage and the associated danger of neglecting to link together the data into a coherent set of interpretations.

It is advocated as a strength of some qualitative software that it enables links to be made to the quantitative world. The package WinMAX, for example, supports the creation of numeric variables from qualitative data for export and further analysis using a statistics package. There is little doubt that such a package assists the integrated approach of qualitative and quantitative analysis tools upon a set of data. However, critics have voiced concern that such software provides no substitute for the conceptual hard work in qualitative analysis. To take an extreme example, if one were to run Shakespeare or Joyce through the software, there would be nothing that the packages could offer in the interpretation of this complex material other than some (probably largely irrelevant) facts about the frequency of occurrence of certain words and themes and their relationship to each other. The understanding of the concepts and ideas behind the imagery, the associations and the descriptions in the texts in their social, historical and cultural contexts and their subsequent interpretation are still 100 per cent up to the human operator.

Thus there is no computer-assisted method available for identifying or extracting themes from textual material other than the rather basic process of searching through text for the frequency of occurrence of certain words and phrases. Given these restrictions, many prefer to adopt the traditional approach to qualitative analysis, using coloured highlighters, pen and paper, and brainpower. They argue that the computer gets in the way of the process of relating to the data.

Having used qualitative software over a number of years, I believe that this is an over-pessimistic position. The computer cannot, of course, produce interpretations of textual material, any more than a statistical analysis package can indicate why different demographic groups have responded differently on an attitudinal questionnaire. These tasks are uniquely human. However, used judiciously and intelligently, the qualitative software can be beneficial. When dealing with a large volume of textual data, the computer can systematise and speed up some of the tedious and complex processes which are necessary preliminaries to reaching interpretations. For example, the package NUD*IST offers the following options, *inter alia*, through its index searching system: the ability to locate passages of text which overlap, appear near, within or never appear alongside other passages of text. An emerging idea or hypothesis about the data, for example that one theme in a set of focus group discussions is normally contingent upon a certain idea or ideas being introduced by other members of the group, can therefore be tested quickly in a systematic way using the features of the index search system. Although, in principle, such a procedure could be achieved manually by reading through the transcripts, identifying relevant passages and collating them as linked piles of paper, this would be extremely laborious if the amount of material was substantial. If the analysis was at an exploratory stage, many such emerging ideas may need to be tested, and in practice, unless the resources of a large team were available, it is unlikely that time and energy would be available to analyse the material in this systematic way. For the lone researcher, therefore, in principle and at best, the software can make tasks associated with the data interpretation achievable which would effectively be impossible through manual methods.

An analogy could be the power that statistical packages bring to bear on the analytic interpretation of numerical data. In principle, a great deal of exploratory regression analyses could be conducted on a dataset, using different combinations of independent variables, by entirely manual methods using a calculator. In practice, the task would be very unlikely to be done, and would be error-prone, because of the complex and lengthy procedures needed to conduct the regression analyses manually. However, this analogy also illustrates an inherent danger in the use of qualitative software. A 'quantitative' approach to content analysis is no substitute for thinking about the data. Whilst the detailed coding and documentation of the text passages may, in some projects, be an aid to its interpretation, no amount of mechanically processing the occurrences of themes and text passages in relation to each other is going to lead to insightful interpretations. Just as the automatic application of statistical analyses to numbers which packages such as SPSS provide will not ensure a correct or meaningful analysis without a thorough understanding of both the data and the tests involved, qualitative analysis needs to be guided at all stages by a thorough grasp of the data in its cultural and interpersonal contexts.

Case study: the analysis of interview transcripts using the WinMAX software

Data for the study described here was kindly provided by Dr Peter Green, Senior Lecturer in Sports Science at University College Chichester. Eight interviews were conducted with staff at a leisure centre in the South of England, as part of a larger study concerned with the effects of management style on the working environment and culture. The first step in the treatment of the data was to transcribe the recorded interviews using a word processor. The data was then saved as an unformatted ASCII file, that is, as files which did not contain any software-specific formatting features. ASCII is an acronym for the American Standard Code for Information Interchange and ASCII files are essentially plain text files which do not have to be accessed by any special software. ASCII files may be produced by word processors using the 'text only with line breaks' option and can also be produced using a text editor such as the one supplied with versions of the Microsoft Windows operating system. ASCII files frequently have the '.txt' file extension.

The study desrcibed here was conducted with two aims: identifying changes in management style since the appointment of a new General Manager some eighteen months previously, and identifying the relationships between management and the working culture of the organisation. The following interviews were carried out with the Leisure Centre staff.

- General Manager
- Heads of Department (two)
- Line managers (two)
- Junior employees (three).

The software used for this analysis was the WinMAX Pro 96 package (there is now a newer version of WinMAX). WinMAX Pro was developed by Dr Udo Kuckartz of the Free University of Berlin. The general scheme of the analysis adopted here was as follows:

1   A new project was started in WinMAX and the ASCII text files imported.
2   Some initial categories (themes) were identified from the thrust of the questions and the answers given.
3   Segments of text were coded against the categories established.
4   The category structure was refined and extended in the light of the ongoing analysis.
5   At various stages memos were written representing interpretations of the data.
6   Text searches were carried out to identify the occurrence of key words.
7   The relationship of the categories to each other was identified as a later stage of the analysis.
8   The report was prepared based upon the memos and the analysis.

The startup screen is shown in Figure 11.1. This screen indicates the main menu system which consists of the following options:

Object select to start a new project, to save projects and files and to print text

Codefunctions provides an index of the coding and the frequencies of codewords

Search to search the text for occurrences of words using logical operators

Variables enables numeric or string variables to be set up and exported

Memos for creating saving and printing memos about the text

Options provides print, save and display options

Help accesses a Windows standard help system

The startup screen shown in Figure 11.1 also indicates the status of the four standard windows associated with WinMAX.

- List of texts
- List of codewords
- List of codings
- Working text.

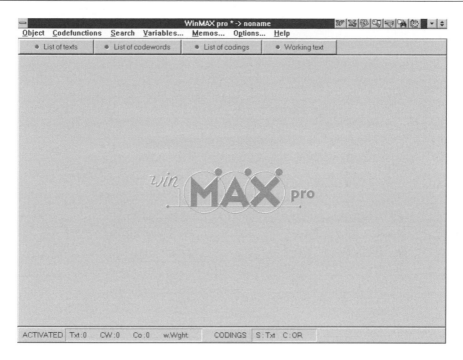

Figure 11.1 Startup screen from WinMAX.

Any of these windows can be turned on or off by pressing the appropriate button. A minimum of one and a maximum of four windows can be simultaneously present to display different information about the data being considered. The 'List of texts' window provides information concerning text files which have been imported and been made available for analysis; the 'List of codewords' window provides a sideways tree diagram of the codewords which have been established and against which individual parts of the text have been assigned. The 'List of codings' window provides a display of all the text, organised by codeword, which has been assigned to each codeword, and the 'Working text' window is a display of the actual text file which has been activated and is being worked upon. WinMAX therefore enables a simultaneous display, for example, of text that is being worked upon (in the 'Working text' window) together with the codewords, or categories, which have been assigned to the text (in the 'List of codewords' window).

In Figure 11.2, the Object: Manager: New menu option was selected to create a new Object which would contain all the interview data and associated coding and analysis for this study. An Object in this context is simply the whole project including all the text files and the associated codewords and memos which will be established. A dialog box is shown where a name for the Object is being specified.

After a new Object had been created, the first stage was to create a new project and to import all the ASCII files consisting of the interview transcripts. A project called 'Leisure centre' was created by clicking with the mouse on the Object filing cabinet in the top left-hand corner of the 'List of texts' window. Text was then imported by clicking on the project icon (a filing cabinet drawer) and choosing the 'Add new text' option. The 'Import text' dialog box

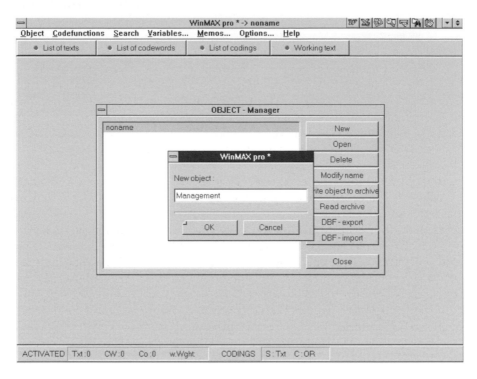

Figure 11.2 Screenshot from WinMAX: specifying Object name.

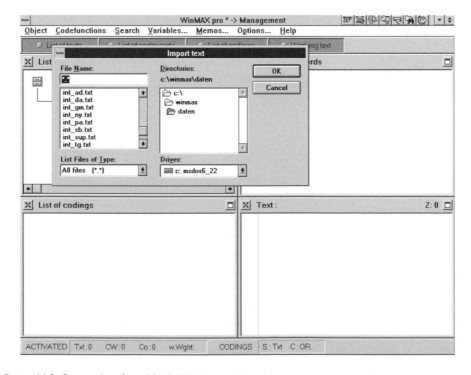

Figure 11.3 Screenshot from WinMAX: importing text.

appeared as is indicated in Figure 11.3, providing a Windows standard way of selecting the drive and directory within which the text files to be imported were residing.

This process is repeated for each text file which you wish to include in the data for analysis. After all the text files have been imported and given a name, one or more can be activated by clicking on the icon for each text file (a page with the top left-hand corner turned down). All the texts appear in the 'List of texts' window with activated texts appearing in a different colour. In the screenshot shown in Figure 11.4, all eight texts which will be used in the analysis have been imported and given a name and the 'General manager' interview text has been activated. The text of this interview therefore appears in the 'Working text' window in the lower right-hand portion of the screen, which can be scrolled upwards and downwards using the Windows standard scroll bars at the edge of the window. In Figure 11.4, the very first part of this interview transcript is displayed.

After all the data in the form of the interview transcripts has been made available in this way, the analysis can begin. The first stage of this analysis was to proceed to coding the text against codewords. That is, units of text from single words to whole paragraphs or more can be assigned to one or more categories, or codewords which may be established. The package cannot assist the process of determining which codewords are appropriate – essentially the codewords are the themes that you determine are present from inspection of the data. The first codeword which was established in this example was one entitled 'Time in post' to indicate how long each employee had been in post, since this related specifically to a question which was asked of each interviewee. The procedure for setting up a new codeword in WinMAX involves clicking on the codeword icon appearing in the 'List of codewords' window and selecting the 'Add new codeword' option. The first piece of coding is shown in Figure 11.5 where, under the 'Time in post' category, the text '2 years' for the General Manager interview has been selected using the left- and right-hand mouse buttons. In WinMAX, text of any length, from a single word to a block of paragraphs, can be selected to code against any pre-defined codeword category. In some other qualitative software packages, the unit of analysis – such as a single line of text – has to be defined in advance.

The process of subsequently assigning this text segment to a codeword is achieved by clicking on the codeword icon and pressing the 'Code' button in the Codeword Manager which appears, as shown in Figure 11.7. Figure 11.6 illustrates a slightly later stage of the coding of these interview texts. The text 'Interview with AD' has been selected (a pencil appears on the icon in the 'List of texts' window) and three lines of text have been selected to be assigned to the 'Time in post' codeword. Figure 11.7 illustrates the Codeword Manager functions. By the stage illustrated in Figure 11.7, some further codewords have been established as follows: 'Dislike about the post' and 'Like about the post'. Text was systematically assigned to each of these codeword categories by reading through and examining the text for each of the eight interviews. That is, the process is essentially a manual one, although it is being conducted with the aid of software. The process of coding the text against each category, or codeword, which has been established can therefore be a slow and exacting process if a great deal of text is involved.

However, the software can offer some shortcuts to this process which may help speed up the analysis. In particular, it is possible to identify all the occurrences of particular words or combinations of words which may be associated with particular categories using the text search capabilities. When the 'Search' menu is selected and the option 'Search' chosen, the dialog box shown in Figure 11.8 appears. Here, all occurrences of the word 'democratic' are being identified in order to assist the process of categorising text against a category

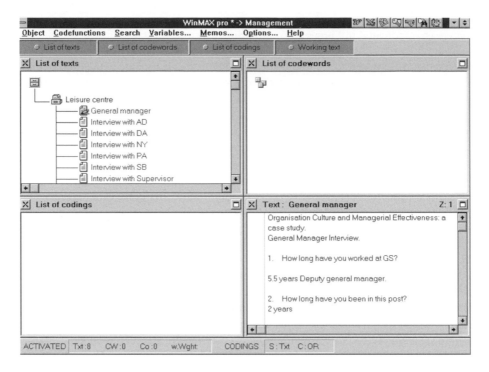

Figure 11.4 Screenshot from WinMAX: activating working text.

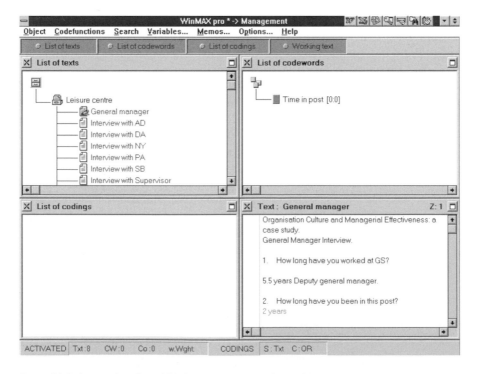

Figure 11.5 Screenshot from WinMAX: procedure for coding.

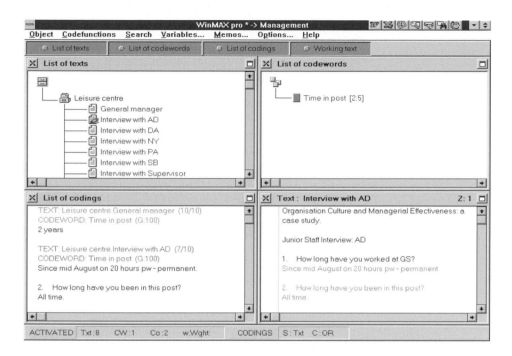

Figure 11.6 Screenshot from WinMAX: assigning text to codeword.

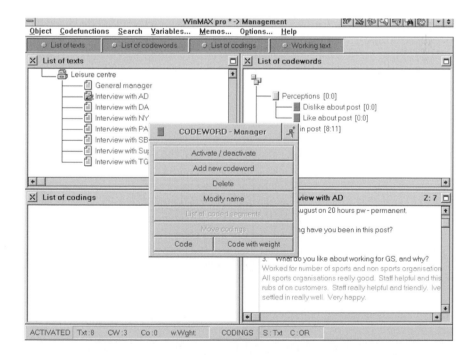

Figure 11.7 Screenshot from WinMAX: Codeword manager functions.

'Management style/democratic'. A search for several words in combination using the OR and the AND operators can also be made.

These text searches may be of benefit if a great deal of text is involved; however, usually it is the concepts and ideas that are important in qualitative analysis rather than the particular words which have been used to express them and the software offers no shortcuts to identifying these. In Figure 11.9, the results of part of the search just described are illustrated. The 'Head of Department1' text has been activated and the window entitled 'Working Text' illustrates an occurrence of the word 'democratic' in the conversation. The 'List of Codings' window shows the text which has been selected and coded against this category. Even if the word 'democratic' has not been used by the particular interviewee, however, it is important that all relevant text in the transcripts is coded against this (or any other) category so the text searching capabilities are only an aid to, and not a substitute for, careful reading through all the text in the 'Working text' window.

It is common practice in qualitative analysis to write notes about the text, the categories which are emerging and their relationship. These notes, or memos, often represent the beginnings of the interpretation of the data. In Figure 11.10, a memo is being created in WinMAX. Memos are used to record any aspect of the interpretation and analysis of the texts. They are thus distinguished from the raw data and can inform the final report of the findings. In this instance, a memo has been created (by clicking with the mouse in the left-hand border in the 'Working text' window) to record the definition of the 'democratic' management style category. In Chapter 10, it was noted how important it was that each category, or codeword in WinMAX terminology, that is established during a qualitative analysis has an associated working definition of what it represents, providing guidelines to enable a decision to be made about the appropriateness of assignation of text in that category. If these definitions are routinely created for each codeword, in principle someone else could come along and repeat your analysis with very similar results.

Figure 11.11 shows the category scheme as it has emerged after several hours of work identifying the codewords and assigning text against them, with two windows which have been made active. The left-hand window indicates the list of texts which are being examined and the right-hand window the list of codewords which have been identified, based around the questions asked and the answers given in the interviews.

Not all the detailed stages concerned with arriving at the keywords identified and illustrated in Figure 11.11 have been worked through in this section. The process is essentially a manual one; that is, reading through the texts and, from the questions asked in the interviews and the ensuing answers given, the themes depicted here have emerged. The process of identifying codewords, or categories, is an iterative one and WinMAX enables the category scheme to be modified in the light of the ongoing analysis of all eight interviews in this case. Although no more than two levels of the ensuing tree structure have been established in Figure 11.11, analyses of more complex material can involve tree structures with three, four or more levels of categories and sub-categories. Establishing these codewords was relatively straightforward as they flowed from the questions asked and the answers recorded in these interviews. In less structured interviews, this may not be the case. The codeword scheme, as has been pointed out in Chapter 10, may be based on a number of different relationships in the material being examined, including logical, aetiological, temporal or other relationships.

Figure 11.12 illustrates part of the output from selecting the 'Codefunctions: Index of codings' menu option. This option is particularly helpful towards the end of the coding process, when you may wish to examine the text in relation to the codewords, for example the

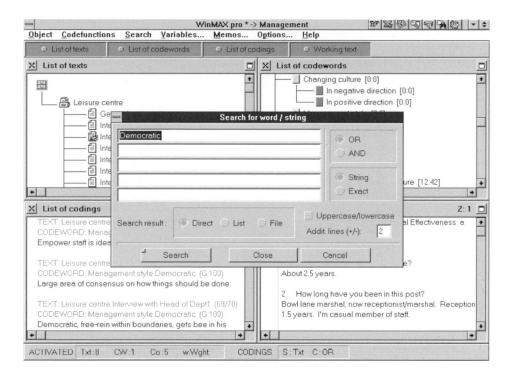

Figure 11.8 Screenshot from WinMAX: searching text.

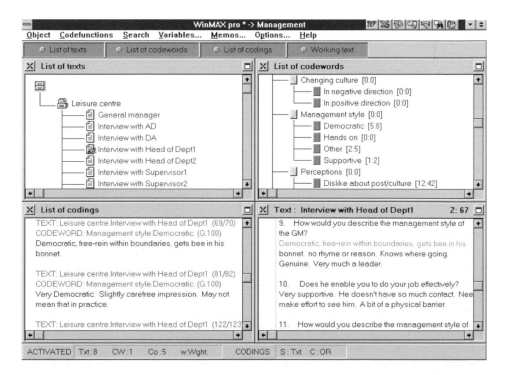

Figure 11.9 Screenshot from WinMAX: result of text search.

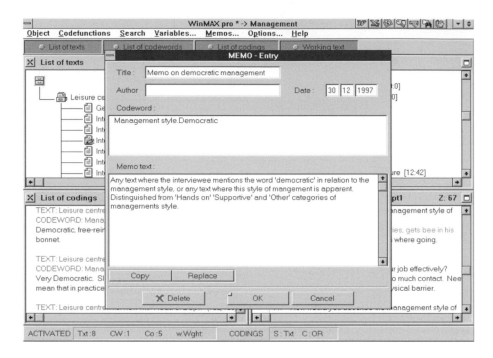

Figure 11.10 Screenshot from WinMAX: creating a memo.

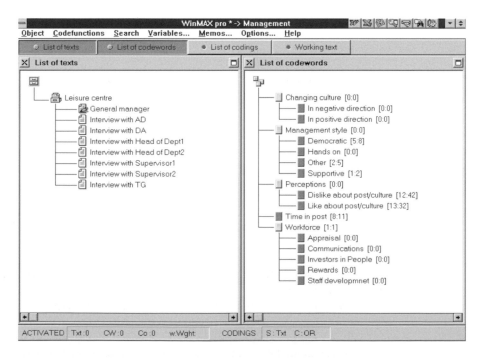

Figure 11.11 Screenshot from WinMAX: category scheme.

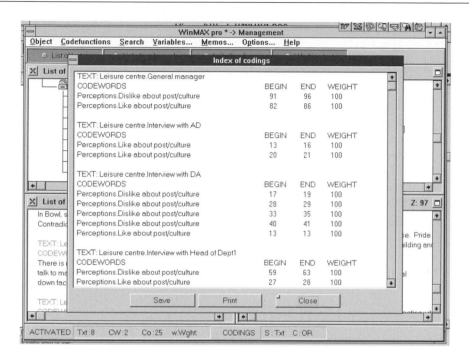

Figure 11.12 Screenshot from WinMAX: Index of codings.

extent to which the text has been completely coded against the themes, the extent of overlaps of the coding (text assigned to more than one category) and so forth. This option therefore provides an overall summary of the coding process. Here, the codewords are listed together with the beginning and ending line numbers for each of the parts of the texts which have been coded against each codeword. The weighting for each of the codings has been chosen as 100 per cent which is the default. WinMAX allows a graded weighting which can be given any percentage value. The weighting function enables a degree of likeness to the ideal characterisation of a concept to be assigned to a segment of text. The weight score can be used to identify the most important segments at a later stage of the analysis. So WinMAX, in addition to permitting 'all or none' coding of text against codewords, allows through the weighting function the degree of relevance of the codeword to a particular piece of text to be subjectively assessed and recorded on a scale of 0–100 per cent.

The final stages of this analysis, therefore, centred upon an examination of the degree to which the codewords which had been assigned adequately reflected the themes in the data, and an examination of the degree to which the categories were, or were not, related to each other through inspection of the 'Index of coding'. The final report which was produced was informed by the various memos which had been created along the way, recording observations and interpretations of the material.

In brief, some overall conclusions from these interviews were that the management style had improved since the appointment of the new General Manager in terms of positive working relationships and the setting of clear goals and objectives. The process of working towards the Investors in People award was generally perceived as valuable by staff with managerial responsibility but little was known about it by junior staff. Overall, there was a perception of a supportive working environment with positive aspects being contact with clients and a generally relaxed working atmosphere; negative aspects included some perceived communication difficulties with senior management and the hassles of getting things done. A final report was therefore written based upon the analyses of these categories of text and the various memos which had been written throughout the process.

The package WinMAX contains other features and capabilities not mentioned here. For example, numeric variables can be set up from the text and exported as .dbf ('dBASE' database standard) files which could then be imported into a statistical analysis package such as SPSS and analysed quantitatively. A newer version of the WinMAX software than the one discussed here has since been made available by Sage Publications. Other qualitative analysis packages provide similar capabilities to the features mentioned here although the way that these are implemented vary. As I have been concerned to emphasise in this book, no qualitative software will provide interpretations of the textual material for you, but used judiciously can assist the process of systematically categorising and analysing the text as a preliminary to reaching conclusions about the data.

Qualitative projects, as much as projects based around quantitative methods, require much background research about the question being approached. Conventional ways of going about this have been augmented in recent years by the information cascade made available through the internet. This is therefore the topic of the next chapter.

Action points

- Decide whether the use of qualitative software will be of assistance to you, bearing in mind the volume of data you have collected, the type of analyses contemplated and the learning curve which may be involved in getting to know the software.
- Work on your analysis and report at the same time; they will inform each other.

Chapter 12

Surfin' safari

What is the internet?

The way that research is conducted clearly changes over time as technical and methodological procedures evolve. Thus traditional academic libraries are fast becoming multi-media information centres, reflected in the name change to 'Learning Resources Centres'. The internet in particular is a new research resource which is changing the way information is located and delivered. What we know as the internet today started out in the 1970s and evolved in the 1980s from the need for computers at academic institutions to link up and communicate with each other, for the exchange of research data, for joint working on projects and so on. Thus the JANET (joint academic network) was born and soon it became possible to link up with academic and commercial computers in the USA, and elsewhere in Europe and the rest of the world. With the explosion of personal computing in the mid- and late 1980s, dial-up access to existing networks of mainframe computers, including the JANET system, through modems attached to the telephone system became more commonplace. In the twenty-first century, the internet today is a huge system of interconnecting networks of computers worldwide. Anybody with a personal computer and modem at home can sign up with an ISP (internet service provider) and access internet resources online. The internet provides the following facilities:

- Access to the world wide web (www) pages
- Access to non-www information such as gopher information
- Access to discussion and newsgroups
- File transfer including downloading of software online (FTP)
- Electronic mail (email).

The best known part of the internet is the world wide web. This is accessed by starting up a 'web browser', which is frequently either the Microsoft Internet Explorer or the Netscape Navigator software. The world wide web is a collection of pages, consisting of text and graphics which provide hypertext links to other pages. The hypertext links are distinguished by colour coding in the text and can be accessed by clicking the mouse on the hypertext words. Thus it is possible to go from one page to another by double clicking on items on pages, ending up at points far distant from the starting place: a process known as 'surfing the net'. Information is available on just about every conceivable subject. Many organisations, businesses and individuals, including every academic institution, each have their own sites. From your starting point, or home page, other sites can be located in one of two ways.

1   If you know the site address you can enter this directly.
2   Search engines and web finders can be used to locate relevant sites.

Thus every site on the internet has its own unique address. For world wide web pages, this is of the form 'http://www.microsoft.com' (the Microsoft home page). In academic reports, there is no universally agreed way of referencing material obtained through the internet. It is, however, good practice to quote the full site address as shown above plus the date when the site was accessed, because sites change from time to time. World wide web addresses of this form appear on many communications from organisations nowadays. It is a good idea to collect your own list of site addresses which might be useful to you. Unfortunately, there are no generally useful 'yellow pages' of addresses where these can be looked up, nor are there any comprehensive directories of email addresses available. To get you started, Appendix II includes some of the most popular health-related sites you may wish to access.

Using search engines

If you do not have a particular site in mind, or do not know its address, one of the search engines can be of assistance in locating relevant information about a topic. This enables you to use alternative web finder and search engine software, including 'Yahoo', 'Infoseek' , 'Lycos' and 'Web Crawler'. It is probably a good idea to get to know one thoroughly, although you may wish to use more than one for a particular search, since they do not each come up with the same results. Infoseek, for example, provides facilities to limit searches to United Kingdom sites only, to search on combinations of words, to search in particular topic areas such as education or health and to limit searches by particular time periods. It is sometimes not appreciated that the search software has a number of built-in advanced searching facilties, which can assist the process of locating relevant and specific information. The 'Infoseek advanced' software is one which I have found meets most search needs. The address of this search software is:

http://infoseek.go.com/find?pg=advanced_www.html&ud9=advanced_www

The following features are built into the 'Infoseek advanced' software.

- Searches can be confined to titles, hyperlinks or whole documents.
- Searches can be carried out on words, phrases or names.
- Searches can be limited to particular sites (such as commercial, government or education).
- Particular countries can be searched as well as the entire web.
- Combinations of words can be searched for simultaneously (AND function).
- Particular words can be excluded (NOT function).

The basic principles of searching the internet using the Infoseek (or similar) software may be summarised as follows:

1   Type one or more words, a name or a short question that defines what you want to search for.
2   Select the set of information within which you wish to search. Dropdown menus are

available below the text entry box to search the whole web or alternatively, for example, to limit the search to a particular country, e.g. the United Kingdom.

3   Press the 'search' or 'seek' button to carry out the search and list the hits. At this point, you can either browse through the hits, or if too many have been generated, the search may be narrowed down, perhaps by entering more specific words or questions.

Unfortunately, none of the software designed to assist the process of searching the web is as sophisticated as we would like. The presently available search engines are all limited, since they fail to take into account the structural links that exist between documents (hypertext links); usually many irrelevant 'hits' are generated by entering a few key words. At the time of writing, a web search engine developed by a team at the Technion–Israeli Institute of Technology offers the way to a future improvement; these researchers have developed a search engine with its own programming language which is able to look for structures or relationships between web documents rather than merely searching for particular words or phrases.

At present, however, the internet is so vast that any general searches, such as on the topics 'dietary advice' or 'skin cancer' are likely to come up with thousands of sites. Many of these are likely to be of marginal relevance at best; locating useful and relevant information on the internet is a challenge in itself. You need always to bear in mind that there are no restrictions on the type or quality of information appearing on the internet – thus anybody can set up web sites and put anything they want on it. The electronic publishing revolution is very democratic! From the academic point of view, information appearing on the internet should thus be treated with a healthy degree of scepticism, unless the source is a recognised reputable organisation, such as the Health Education Authority, the National Library of Medicine or whatever. Information which has been obtained from the internet may be used and referenced in student work in much the same way as information appearing in journals and books, with the above caveat in mind. If this is done, the full site address needs to be given in the reference to enable someone else to locate it, in the same way as the author, the publisher and so on would be given for a printed reference.

Perhaps the greatest strength of using the internet in this way, to locate background information for a research project, is that it provides much information not readily available anywhere else. Thus, if the project is about 'skin cancer', for example, you would, of course, carry out conventional scientific literature searches using the MEDLINE, CINAHL and other databases that are available. However, much other information not appearing in printed form is available on this topic. This is the area known as 'grey literature'.

One particular search for example on the term 'malignant melanoma' produced over 3,000 'hits', the first part of which contained the following.

Search > +"malignant melanoma"

Search results

3,234 matches   Next 10 > | Hide summaries | Sort by date | Ungroup results

1. Cancer control Journal: Accurate Nodal Staging of Malignant Melanoma
Cutaneous Oncology Program at H. Lee Moffitt Cancer Center & Research Institute, Tampa, Fla. The incidence of malignant melanoma is increasing at a faster pace than ...
Relevance: 91% Date: 18 Mar 1999, Size 48.7K,
 http://www.moffitt.usf.edu/cancjrnl/v2n5/article4.html
Find similar pages | Translate this page

2. The Melanoma Project
THE MALIGNANT MELANOMA PROJECT Introduction The occurrence of malignant melanoma (cancer in birthmarks) is rapidly rising. In Denmark the figure has more than 10-folded during the last 50 years. In the ...
Relevance: 90% Date: 27 Oct 1999, Size 3.7K,
 http://ei.dtu.dk/staff/hintz/WWW/Melanoma/melanoma.html
Find similar pages | Translate this page

3. Funny Moles and Malignant Melanoma Information page - The Little Surgery, Stamford, UK
A patient information leaflet - Funny Moles and Malignant Melanoma. This is one of a series of information leaflets available on The Little Surgery, Stamford, ...
Relevance: 82% Date: 18 Dec 1998, Size 13.4K,
 http://web.ukonline.co.uk/ruth.livingstone/little/melanoma.htm
Find similar pages | Translate this page

4. dotPHARMACY:update malignant melanoma
To appreciate the HEA's sun care message To distinguish between malignant melanoma
and other skin cancers To be familiar with the appearance of a malignant melanoma To be aware of the pharmacist's ...
Relevance: 80%   Date: 16   Jun   1997,   Size   10.2K,
http://www.dotpharmacy.co.uk/uptan.html
Find similar pages | More results from www.dotpharmacy.co.uk | Translate this page

5. superficial spreading malignant melanoma
The edge of the right upper quadrant of this lesion is remarkable for the difference in color from the remainder of the lesion. Note how most of the tumor is brown and tan, whereas ...
Relevance: 79% Date: 5 Aug 1998, Size 8.0K,
 http://matrix.ucdavis.edu/tumors/tradition/gallery-ssmm.html
Find similar pages | More results from matrix.ucdavis.edu | Translate this page

6. Malignant Melanoma Fact Sheet

Q. What is malignant melanoma? A. Malignant melanoma, a very serious skin cancer, is characterized by the uncontrolled growth of pigment-producing tanning cells. Melanomas may suddenly appear without ...

Relevance: 76% Date: 7 May 1999, Size 7.8K,

 http://www.aad.org/SkinCancerNews/magmel.htm

Find similar pages | More results from www.aad.org | Translate this page

7. PPP healthcare International-Health Info-MALIGNANT MELANOMA

MALIGNANT MELANOMA What is it? The cells in the skin which cause tanning of the skin in response to sunlight are called melanocytes. Sometimes these cells can ...

Relevance: 74% Date: 29 Jul 1999, Size 13.4K,

 http://www.ppphealthcare.co.uk/html/health/melanoma.htm

Find similar pages | Translate this page

8. Disease Category Listing (196): Malignant Melanoma

CenterWatch Listing of Clinical Research Trials for Malignant Melanoma

Relevance: 73% Date: 10 Dec 1999, Size 6.5K,

 http://www.centerwatch.com/studies/cat196.htm

Find similar pages | Translate this page

9. FDA Clears Intron A as an Adjuvant Therapy for Malignant Melanoma

MADISON, N.J., Dec. 6, 1995 -- Schering-Plough Corporation (NYSE: SGP) today announced clearance by the Food and Drug Administration of INTRON(R) A (Interferon alfa-2b, recombinant) for ...

Relevance: 73%   Date: 21   Mar   1996,   Size   5.7K,
http://www.pslgroup.com/dg951207a.htm

Find similar pages | More results from www.pslgroup.com | Translate this page

10. Malignant Melanoma

MALIGNANT MELANOMA Synonyms Melanoma Melanocarcinoma Overview Malignant melanoma (MM) is a malignant neoplasm of epidermal melanocytes. Melanoma is the third most common skin cancer and represents ...

Relevance: 73% Date: 21 Sep 1998, Size 31.0K,

 http://www.dentalcare.com/soap/intermed/melan.htm

Find similar pages | Translate this page

This particular web search has come up with access to a listing of clinical trials on the topic, diagnostic information and information on the malignant melanoma project. These site descriptions provide a way in to further information on each topic, using the hypertext links, which are blue on screen and shown here in grey. This search was too general and many of the three thousand or more hits were of little relevance. The researcher was actually interested in health promotion activities around malignant melanoma. A more specific search was therefore carried out using the Infoseek advanced software to confine the search to sites where 'malignant melanoma' appeared in the title and 'health promotion' appeared in the document. This produced a much more restricted listing including a consensus statement from the US National Institute of Health on the primary and secondary prevention of the disease. This was referenced by the researcher in her report as follows:

> NIH (1992) What is the role of education and screening in preventing melanoma morbidity and mortality? National Institute of Health Consensus Statements 88: Diagnosis and Treatment of Early Melanoma.
> http://odp.od.nih.gov/consensus/cons/088/088_statement.htm#6_What_Is
> Accessed January 2000

You will often find that, in order to access some software feature or file type, a particular additional piece of software, known as a 'plugin' is required. Plugins can be downloaded from internet sites and a message will generally appear in the browser when this is necessary. Many text files, for example, are presented on the world wide web as PDF (portable document format) files and you will need to download the Adobe Acrobat reader software to access their information. The PDF files provide a way of displaying documents which are independent of the computer platform being used.

   Data available through the internet could be used as the basis itself for research projects. Thus a set of national databases of statistics is available, for example, at The University of Essex site, containing ESRC and other research material which are publicly available as national databases. Information from these archives can thus be downloaded, using the file transfer protocol (FTP) and analysed offline. Worthy of particular mention is the National Electronic Library for Health (NELH) which became available in prototype form towards the end of 1999. The purpose of this national resource created by the NHS Information Authority is to provide ready access to the best available knowledge to assist practice and patient care. It is informed by a multitude of sources including information from the National Institute of Clinical Excellence (NICE) and the NHS Research and Development programme, and the library has access to standard medical databases such as MEDLINE.

Case study: using the Cochrane database

The Cochrane library is a resource widely used by professional health researchers. The Cochrane database of systematic reviews (CDSR) provides the findings of meta-analyses of published studies on the effects of health care, mainly of randomised controlled trials. The library also provides access to a database of abstracts of reviews of effectiveness (DARE) which have been subject to appraisal by the NHS Centre for Reviews and Dissemination at the University of York. The MRC clinical trials register is also available through the Cochrane library. Full access to the Cochrane material is available only by subscription but the abstracts of Cochrane reviews can be browsed and searched by anyone with internet access. The use of

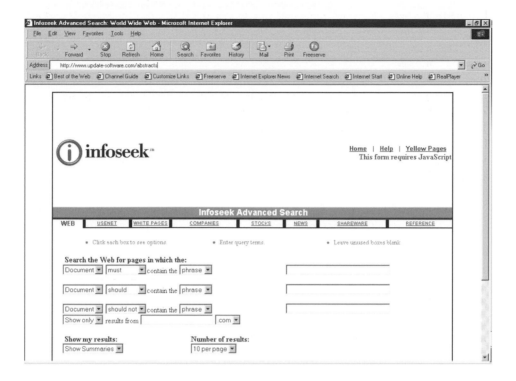

Figure 12.1 Screenshot from Infoseek search software.

Note

the Cochrane reviews can be illustrated by a case study of a medical student who needed to obtain an up-to-date summary of best evidence on the effectiveness of the drug Donepezil in the treatment of people with Alzheimer-type dementia. The student, who was writing an assignment on the treatment of degenerative brain conditions by substances which modify the effects of neurotransmitters, used the Cochrane database to locate a meta-analysis of published studies on this drug.

The site address of the Cochrane abstracts was entered in the web browser (see Figure 12.1). It is:

http://www.update-software.com/abstracts/

This takes us directly to the Cochrane abstracts search engine as is shown in Figure 12.2. At this point, the search term of interest – Donepezil – was entered and the screen shown in Figure 12.3 appeared.

The option 'Cochrane dementia and cognitive impairment group abstracts' was selected from the screen shown in Figure 12.3, producing the information shown in Figure 12.4.

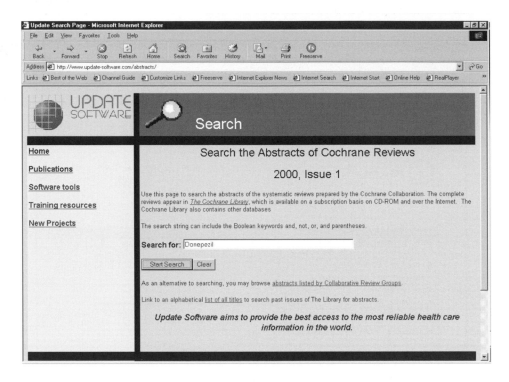

Figure 12.2 Screenshot from Cochrane database: search item entered.

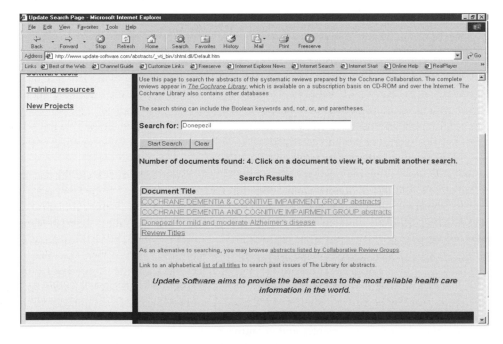

Figure 12.3 Screenshot from Cochrane database: result of search.

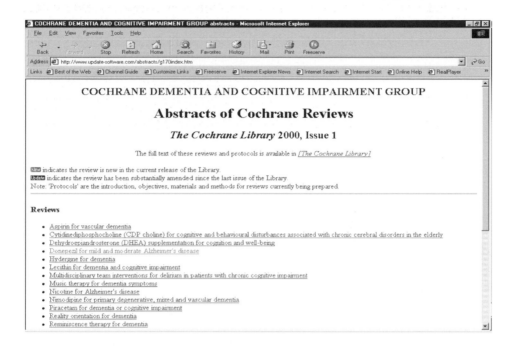

Figure 12.4 Screenshot from Cochrane database: abstract selected.

The Donepezil review was then selected producing the abstract which is shown on pp. 118–119.

The review abstract indicates the evidence upon which it was based; a search of standard databases and clinical trials directories produced four relevant studies which were reviewed. The conclusions are summarised from the meta-analysis of these studies. The Cochrane library is a major example of the ideology, which gained momentum in the 1990s and is consolidating in the early part of the twenty-first century, that health care delivery should be firmly rooted in the principles of evidence-based methods and practice. This ideology has stemmed, in the UK, as much from the practical need to contain budgets within the NHS as from a philosophical commitment to a quantitative approach to the evaluation of evidence on the effectiveness of health care interventions.

In the Donepezil review shown above, for example, the selection criteria for the review were 'all unconfounded, double-blind, randomised controlled trials ...'. The comments made on the limitations of RCTs in Chapter 3 should be borne in mind in the evaluation of the review. It is pertinent to note, for example, that despite the findings of the review some modest improvements in cognitive function were evident as a result of the drug that 'the patient's own rating of their quality of life showed no benefit of Donepezil...' and further, that 'there were significantly more withdrawals before the end of treatment from the 10mg/day Donepezil group ...'. These statements might provide clues to a qualitative researcher to follow up a line of enquiry that any perceived benefits of the treatment in relation to disadvantages might not be at all evident from the patients' point of view.

Donepezil for mild and moderate Alzheimer's disease

Birks J S, Melzer D

ABSTRACT

A substantive amendment to this systematic review was last made on 21 August 1998. Cochrane reviews are regularly checked and updated if necessary.

Background: Alzheimer's disease is the most common cause of dementia and is a primary degenerative disease of the brain of unknown cause. Onset is usually late in life with increasing impairment of memory, developing gradually into a global impairment of cognition, orientation, linguistic ability and judgement. The clinical course is accompanied by growing disability and dependency on care. One of the characteristic features of the disease is the widely variable rate of progression seen in different patients.

Acetylcholine is an important neurotransmitter associated with memory, and abnormalities in cholinergic neurones (including cell loss) are among the many neurological and neurochemical abnormalities that develop in AD. One approach to lessening the impact of these abnormalities is to inhibit the breakdown of acetylcholine by blocking the relevant enzyme. Tacrine was the first compound approved as a treatment for AD in the US and worked in this way, but caused severe side effects. E2020 (donepezil, Aricept) is a second generation cholinesterase inhibitor and appears to be highly specific, with relatively few side effects.

Objectives: The objective of this review is to assess whether or not donepezil improves the well-being of patients with mild or moderate Alzheimer's disease.

Search strategy: The Cochrane Dementia and Cognitive Impairment Group Register of Clinical Trials, was searched using the terms 'donepezil', 'E2020' and 'ARICEPT'.

Medline, PsychLIT and EMBASE electronic databases were searched with the above terms. Members of the Donepezil Study Group and Eisai Inc were contacted.

Selection criteria: All unconfounded, double-blind, randomised controlled trials in which treatment with donepezil was administered for more than a day and compared with placebo in patients with Alzheimer's disease.

Data collection and analysis: Data were extracted independently by the reviewers (JSB & DB), pooled where appropriate and possible, and the weighted or standardised mean differences or Peto odds ratios (95%CI) estimated. Where possible, intention-to-treat data were used.

Main results: There are 4 included trials, covering treatment of 12 or 24 weeks duration in highly selected patients. The only information available on one trial (Gauthier 1998) is a conference abstract which reports no usable results. Available outcome data cover domains including cognitive function and global clinical state, but data on several important dimensions of outcome are not available.

The results of three trials suggest a small beneficial effect of donepezil in improving cognitive function: at a 5mg/day dose, improvements measured -2.6 points (95%CI -3.5 — -1.8) on weighted mean difference, in the midrange of the 70 point ADAS-Cog scale. The results of two trials show some improvement in global clinical state (assessed by an independent clinician) in those treated with donepezil compared to placebo. The patient's own rating of their Quality of Life showed no benefit of donepezil compared with placebo. There were significantly more withdrawals before the end of treatment from the 10mg/d (but not the 5mg/d) donepezil group compared with placebo, which may have resulted in some overestimation of beneficial changes at 10mg/d in progressively declining characteristics, as last available measures were used in analyses.

A variety of adverse effects were recorded, but very few patients left a trial as a direct result of the intervention.

Reviewers' conclusions: In selected patients with mild or moderate Alzheimer's disease treated for periods of 12 or 24 weeks, donepezil produced modest improvements in cognitive function and study clinicians rated global clinical state more positively in treated patients. No improvements were present on patient self-assessed quality of life and data on many important outcomes are not available. The practical importance of these changes to patients and carers is unclear.

Citation: Birks J S, Melzer D. Donepezil for mild and moderate Alzheimer's disease (Cochrane Review). In: *The Cochrane Library,* Issue 1, 2000. Oxford: Update Software.

This is an abstract of a regularly updated, systematic review prepared and maintained by the Cochrane Collaboration. The full text of the review is available in *The Cochrane Library* (ISSN 1464-780X).

See or contact Update Software, for information on subscribing to *The Cochrane Library* in your area.

Update Software Ltd, Summertown Pavilion, Middle Way, Oxford OX2 7LG, UK (Tel:+44 1865 513902; Fax:+44 1865 516918)

Other useful health sites

The Department of Health (DoH) site is another valuable resource for the health researcher. It includes databases of health service circulars, published and grey literature reports, details from health surveys, national health statistics and press releases, all of which can be downloaded and printed out as required. The DoH supports the National Research Register (NRR) which is a list of over 50,000 recently completed and currently ongoing research studies within the NHS, many of which have not reached the stage of publication. The type of information available on these ongoing research studies is illustrated in the following record which provides information about a primary care study being conducted within the BHB Community Health Care NHS Trust.

Involving children and their families in implementing integrated and effective care for children in primary care

Lead researcher

BHB Community Care NHS Trust
Bentley Suite, St George's Hospital
117 Suttons Lane
Hornchurch Essex
RM12 6RS

Principal research question

The project aims to involve children and their families in addition to primary health care teams in the implementation of research evidence to improve child health in Barking and Havering and generate widespread understanding of the application of research evidence in primary care

Methodology description

Questionnaires, Focus groups

Sample group description

Children (and their families) treated at GP practices in Barking and Havering HA

Outcome measure description

Data from topic* audits
Observation notes and records from each focus group
Hospital activity data in the selected topic areas

*Topics to be agreed between practices and the project's Steering Group from the following list:

adenoids and tonsillectomy
circumcision
detection of undetected testes
asthma
epilepsy
head injury
glue ear
appropriate antibiotic prescribing
management of upper respiratory tract infection
management of otitis media, conjunctivitis and gastroenteritis
management of urinary tract infection
effective health promotion for teenage mothers

Project status

Ongoing

Funding Information

Funding organisation name: NHS Executive London
Funding reference number: 985

Primary keywords

MeSH terms not yet assigned

NRR data provider

NHS Executive London Region: London Regional Office

The National Research Register

The NRR also contains details of the Medical Research Council's Clinical Trials Register and reviews collated by the NHS Centre for Reviews and Dissemination.

The Bath Information Data Service (BIDS) is a valuable academic resource for the researcher. Ingenta is a company formed through a partnership with the University of Bath, and Ingenta Journals provides access to full-text articles from some 2,500 academic and professional journals to journal subscribers. However, abstracts can be searched and viewed online without charge and BIDS also provides access to the MEDLINE database.

The United States National Library of Medicine (NLM) has had a policy for several years of providing a number of searchable international medical databases available through the internet free of charge. These include:

- Aidsline – HIV literature
- Bioethicsline – medical ethics

- Cancerlit – oncology literature
- Healthstar – health services research
- Hstat – full text clinical guidelines and technology assessments
- Medline – general medical, dental, nursing and pre-clinical sciences
- Medlineplus – consumer health information.

These databases can be fully searched, and referencing information and summaries of articles viewed, printed or saved to disk. Although very many databases are available online, as indicated above, and a vast resource of grey literature is at the researcher's fingertips through the web, commercial considerations do limit the availability of much valuable research information. Thus, although all the recognised journals have web sites and may provide lists of contents and summaries of articles, the full text of many published journals is generally not available online unless subscriptions to the printed versions have been taken out. Your academic library, if it subscribes, may be able to provide a password to access the information. For similar reasons, the content of most printed books is not accessible online, although in the future this is likely to change. Trends in this direction include the publishing of academic research articles and books electronically by individuals as an alternative to traditional methods of publishing. A major advantage of this is the fast and accurate search and location available and the hypertext links to background material. Having said this, there is, of course, no substitute for 'hard copy' that can be carried around in the briefcase and read at any time. The first thing that many researchers do after locating relevant sites is to print out the contents and – whether out of habit or not – many people prefer to work from the printed word on paper than to scroll up and down through screenfuls of information.

Newsgroups

The internet also provides a way for individuals with special research or other interests to communicate with others throughout the world, via forums or discussion groups held online. The internet facilities are a valuable addition to information services; learn how to use the system effectively to improve your research. Like all research, doing your 'homework' before accessing the world wide web pages will pay dividends. Think about the information you need and ways of obtaining it. If you want information on 'the brain' but the information is likely to be too general or non-specific, then some more technically specific words like 'caudate nucleus', 'hypothalamus' or 'corpus callosum' might point the search in the right direction.

Newsgroups can also be an efficient way of finding specific facts. Posting a message to the right newsgroup usually brings a sensible and expert answer. There are newsgroups on every possible subject, but do not contact a newsgroup until you are sure it is the right place to ask your questions. A list of FAQs, that is, Frequently Asked Questions, is likely to be available and ensure that you do not annoy people by asking the same question as everybody else. Asking the same question to several relevant newsgroups at the same time is also frowned upon, since the same people are likely to subscribe to them.

Putting material on the web

Many researchers nowadays are making summaries of findings available on world wide web pages, as was illustrated in the melanoma material in this chapter. All world wide web material exists in the form of 'HTML' (hypertext markup language) files which can be produced by an HTML editor or by many other packages including some word processors. Newer versions of Microsoft Word, for example, provide an option to save text files in web language, including the insertion of hypertext links. These files can then be electronically downloaded as web pages, assuming you have an Internet Service Provider which provides you with web space. If you think you may need to do this, you are referred to one of the specialised texts dealing with web page design and the use of HTML files. A great deal of information on web design is also available online, of course, and the following site may be useful to get you started:

http://www.atwebsites.com/contents.html

Action points

- Become familiar with the browser and search software.
- Save items as text or html files as you find them and sort them out later.
- Make notes about where you've been, carefully recording site addresses.
- Build up your collection of useful internet site addresses for future use.

Chapter 13

Writing your proposal

It may seem strange at this point in the book to be reading about writing your project proposal, because you will be doing this before any research is carried out. I would hope, however, that the previous chapters have been part of your preparation towards this end. Before you actually carry out any research – apart from preliminary work such as literature searching – you will need to state to supervisors and other interested parties exactly what you hope to achieve in the project and how it will be carried out. Although requirements differ in various places, a research proposal need not be a lengthy document, perhaps 2000 words or so. The structure of a typical research proposal would include the following:

- Working title for the project
- The research question(s) being addressed
- Brief summary of relevant previous work in the field
- Reasons for undertaking the research
- Aims of the research
- The methods you intend to use
- The resources required
- Intended outcomes and plans for dissemination of findings
- A timetable for the study
- A short list of key references.

Although a succinctly written document, a research proposal should include enough detail to enable a supervisor or others whose approval you may require to assess the merits of what you wish to do. The aims should therefore be clear; two or three specific aims for a study is usually enough and the aims should not be over-ambitious. Remember that the extent to which the aims are achieved will be used as a yardstick to measure the success of the project. The aims will flow from the specific research question that you are addressing, which should be stated in the proposal. The research question should not be too vague and general or too big to be properly addressed, for example, 'Is religious belief beneficial to health?' A more specific research question that could conceivably be addressed in a student project around this issue, perhaps through a comparative survey, might be: 'Do churchgoers in Littletown have a healthier lifestyle than atheists?'

The research question in turn should flow from the previous work in the field that you have identified through preliminary literature searches. Thus sufficient research evidence has been published reasonably to support a hypothesis that, controlling for age and social class variables, people who go to church tend, for example, to use less alcohol, tobacco and other drugs.

You might come to the conclusion, however, that the evidence is not strong and the reason you feel the research project is justified is that there is room for further investigation in this field and no studies have been published on the specific question you wish to address.

The methods that you intend to use to address the research question should be stated. In the above example, you would need to state how the churchgoers and the atheists were to be identified, how they would be matched for age and social class and how the information on lifestyle was to be obtained. If a previously validated questionnaire instrument is to be used, a reference to this should be included. How is the questionnaire to be distributed and returned to the researcher? The size of the sample to be used is an important statement in a proposal: are the numbers likely to be enough to answer the question of interest? Is your estimate of the required sample size based on preliminary work?

The methods of analysis should also be stated, although it is appreciated in a proposal that a general scheme of analysis is all that may be firmly stated in advance. The intention to submit a study to an ethics committee needs to be stated in a proposal, as do any actions taken to protect confidentiality.

Resources required successfully to carry out a project should be stated – resources including time, collaboration from others, expert advice on analysis, equipment and so forth, in addition to money. Those who look at a proposal will examine the proposed study in relation to the overall time and resources available to complete it. You need to lay out a realistic timescale for each major activity in the project – such as literature searching, contacting a sample, distributing questionnaires, analysing and reporting the findings. Finally, a proposal should say something about your plans to communicate findings to respondents, to other agencies and for publication if appropriate.

A research proposal should be a very carefully researched and written document and every word in it should count. It is not the place systematically to review literature – that is left to your project report – although you need to communicate that you are generally aware of the state of play of research in the field. It is a working document upon which decisions will be made about the viability of your research plans and is worth the expenditure of considerable thought and effort. Most of all, putting your research plans on paper will benefit you, by concentrating and crystallising your thinking on the design of the study.

Colin Robson lists ten ways to get a proposal turned down; this nicely summarises much of the message.

> Don't follow the directions or guidelines for your kind of proposal. Omit information that is asked for. Ignore word limits.
>
> Ensure that the title has little relationship to the stated objectives, and that neither title nor objectives link to the proposed methods or techniques.
>
> Produce woolly, ill-defined objectives.
>
> Have the statement of the central problem or research focus vague, or obscure it by other discussion.
>
> Leave the design and methodology implicit; let them guess.
>
> Have some mundane task, routine consultancy or poorly conceptualized data trawl masquerade as a research project.
>
> Be unrealistic in what can be achieved with the time and resources you have available.

Be either very brief, or, preferably long-winded and repetitive in your proposal. Rely on weight rather than quality.

Make it clear what the findings of your research are going to be, and demonstrate how your ideological stance makes this inevitable.

Don't worry about a theoretical or conceptual framework for your research. You want to do a down-to-earth study so you can forget all that fancy stuff.

(Robson 1993:468)

Action points

- Identify published papers on your chosen topic.
- Discuss your ideas with supervisors and peers.
- Keep your proposal clear and succinct.

Chapter 14

Carrying out a research project

The collection and analysis of your data essentially occupies the bulk of the time you will devote to your project. This will include further reading, laboratory or field data collection and the analysis of your findings. Literature searching is best accomplished using CD-ROM and online facilities which are widely available in academic and medical libraries. These may include the following databases.

- CINAHL (Nursing literature)
- ASSIA (Social Sciences)
- SPORTDISCUS (Sports and exercise physiology)
- Social Trends (Demographic and other statistics)
- PSYCHLIT (Psychological literature)
- CLINPSYC (Clinical psychology)
- MEDLINE (Medical, Biomedical, Dental and Nursing literature).

In recent times, the internet has expanded the possibilities for gaining access to much background and grey literature material which may be of relevance to a study, as has been discussed in Chapter 12.

Searching the literature

A comprehensive literature search is an important early step in conducting a project, and you will be expected to cite all important relevant papers in your final report. You do not, of course, have to identify and read all relevant papers before starting to collect your own data. Do not worry unduly if the topic you have chosen does not throw up many relevant references: you may be working on an original topic which has not been over-researched. Before coming to this conclusion, however, make sure that you have conducted the search properly. As illustrated below, MEDLINE and many other databases are indexed according to a standard set of terms, the MeSH (Medical Subject Headings scheme). The system is American in origin so that if you search on 'general practitioners' or 'cancer' you will only pick up references which happen to mention these terms in the article, whereas if you search on 'physicians, family', and 'neoplasms' which are indexed terms, you will pick up many more articles. The lesson is to use the online thesaurus and indexing systems to get your search terms correct. One difficulty with identifying literature through the use of international databases such as MEDLINE is that many articles identified are published in obscure journals that are difficult to obtain.

Inevitably this means use of the inter-library loans (ILL) system to obtain articles not available in local academic or medical libraries.

Case study: A CD-ROM literature search

WinSPIRS is the Silverplatter Information Retrieval System; it is widely used software which will help you to search and locate references from databases including the CINAHL (Cumulative Index of Nursing and Allied Health), MEDLINE (online Index Medicus) and PSYCHLIT (Psychological Abstracts) products. These databases, along with many others available through Silverplatter and other providers, provide a rapid and comprehensive way of conducting a literature search, both prior to conducting a research study and when writing a literature review for a project report.

The initial steps in conducting a search centre on determining the most relevant keywords to initiate the search. You need to balance the danger of being too general, which will generate many 'hits' (retrieved records) not relevant to your topic, with the other extreme of being too specific, perhaps by using a complex and unusual phrase.

The case study illustrated here outlines the steps and search strategy used by a health studies student who wished to locate published papers concerning a serious form of skin cancer (malignant melanoma) and, in particular, to find studies which were concerned with health promotion strategies in respect of this increasingly prevalent disease. The term 'malignant melanoma' has been entered on the 'Search' line using a 1997 MEDLINE disk and WinSPIRS. The screenshot shown in Figure 14.1 indicates the result.

Below the search area seen in Figure 14.1 is the search history area. The search history tracks each search that you carry out. At the moment, it is indicating that one search term, 'malignant melanoma', has been entered and this has produced 303 records containing the term. Consecutive searches are assigned consecutive search numbers. Below the history area is the retrieved records area. By default, all records are displayed with basic referencing information, including details of authors, title, publication year and place of publication. The 'All fields' button at the bottom of the screen can be pressed to display all indexed fields, including abstracts if these are present.

To the left of each record displayed is a symbol: click on this symbol to select particular records for printing or saving to disk. By default, a search on the entered term is carried out across all fields and records in the database. There are, however, field-specific indexes available by pressing the index button and entering a term to look up in the index. On the Utilities menu, there is also an option to choose 'Fields to search' which can provide the option, for example, to limit searches to terms appearing in the titles of articles. In the following example shown in Figure 14.2, the term 'melanoma' has been located in the index and this indicates that a total of 1203 records on this disk contain the term and a total of 4786 occurrences of the word arise in these records.

Although it is not shown in a screenshot in this case study, it is possible to enter various operators to limit the selection of records produced in a search. For example, if 'robertson in au' is entered on the Search line, this command will search for all occurrences of the name Robertson appearing in the 'author' field of the records. Similarly, if 'england in cp' is entered, this will limit the search to articles where the country of publication (the 'cp' field) is England. The use of the following operators can also be employed in searches.

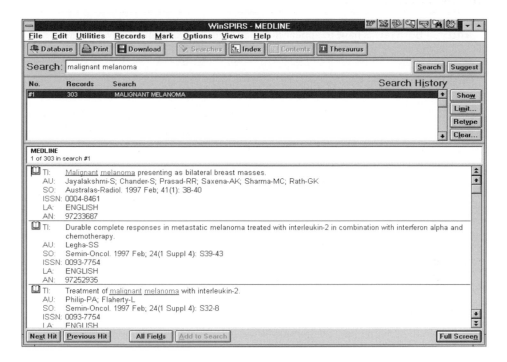

Figure 14.1 Screenshot of MEDLINE references in WinSPIRS.

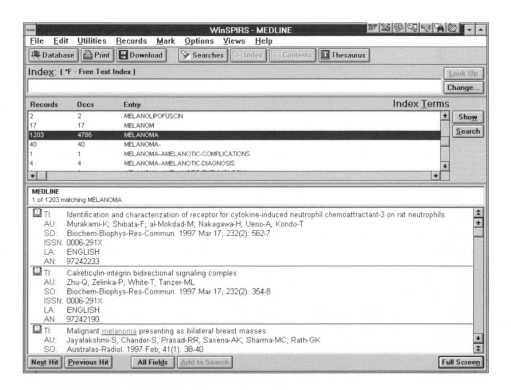

Figure 14.2 Screenshot of MEDLINE references: field-specific index.

and   Both terms have to appear in the record. This option narrows a search down.

or   One or other (or both) terms must appear in the record. This broadens a search.

with   Both terms have to appear in the same field. This narrows a search even further.

near   Both terms have to appear in the same sentence.

not   The first term should appear but not the second in the same record.

Searches such as the above frequently generate a large number of records, many of which may not be relevant to your purposes. The 'Limit' button, which appears to the right of 'Search history' area (see Figure 14.1) is another way of confining a search, for example by country of publication or year of publication, to terms appearing only in the title of an article or to a review article only. In the example shown in Figure 14.3, the limit being selected is that the term should appear in a literature review article.

The thesaurus can also be used to carry out more specific searches. This is accessed by pressing the 'Thesaurus' button which appears on the toolbar; subsequently a dialog box appears and terms may be entered and looked up. In Figure 14.4, part of the thesaurus for this database is displayed. In the MEDLINE thesaurus, a tree of terms is displayed and searches may be narrowed by selecting specific branches of the tree.

This search on malignant melanoma was too general for the purpose of the researcher. The researcher was actually interested in health promotion in relation to the topic. A second search was therefore carried out by entering in the Search line: 'health near (promotion or education)' in order to locate articles where the terms 'health promotion' or 'health education' appeared. These terms were first checked as being in the permuted index. Consecutive searches carried out are given a number preceded by the hash sign (#): the first search is #1, the second #2, and so on. This is a shorthand method of repeating or combining search terms in various ways. In this case, the health studies student made the search more specific to the

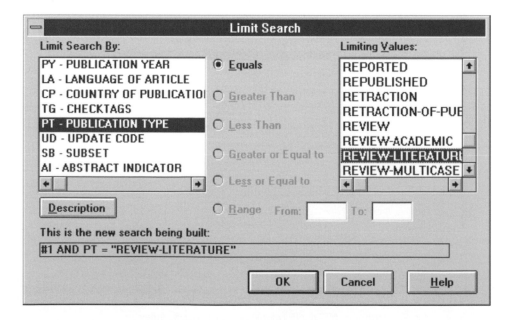

Figure 14.3 Screenshot from WinSPIRS: limiting the search.

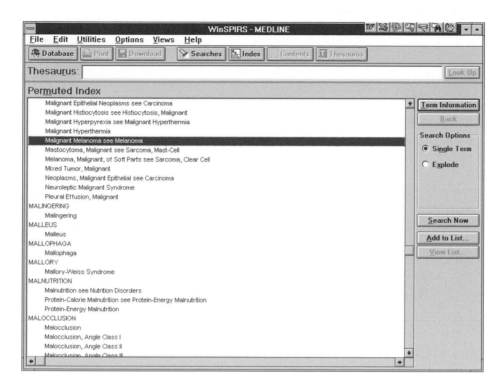

Figure 14.4 Screenshot from WinSPIRS: thesaurus.

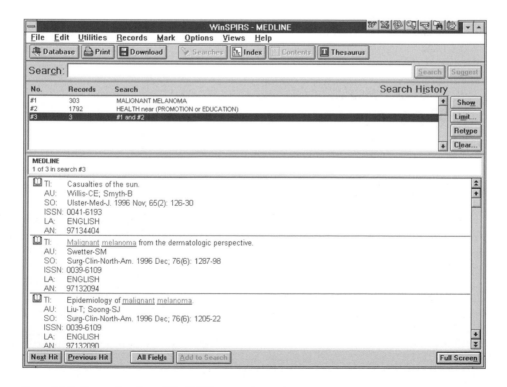

Figure 14.5 Screenshot from WinSPIRS: second search.

objectives of her study by entering on the search line as the third search '#1 and #2' in order to confine the search to records concerned with health promotion or education aspects of malignant melanoma. This narrowed the search down to three specific references in that year, as illustrated in Figure 14.5.

Once you are sure you have located relevant references using combinations of the above techniques, the 'hits' may be printed directly or, more frequently, saved to disk for incorporation into a database of references or for printing out at a later stage. Either all retrieved records or those that have been marked, as indicated above, may be printed or saved. The output to disk is a standard ASCII text file, that is, a file which does not contain any software-specific formatting features. This file may be imported into a text editor or word processor, or into many database management systems. If you wish to print out or save abstracts along with the basic referencing information, do not forget to select the 'All fields' button at the search screen. Search histories may also be saved, and this is a valuable feature if you wish to repeat specific searches exactly the same way each time, perhaps on a monthly basis as the latest references become available.

Databases such as MEDLINE are issued on disks one year at a time and a comprehensive search may need to go back five or more years. Once you have refined your search strategy on one year, you will need to change disks and press the 'Database' button on the toolbar to bring up a dialog box to enable you to access other years and re-run your search history over the new years. A little used feature in my experience is the option on the 'Records' menu to 'Sort records'. This facility provides options to sort hits in ascending or descending order, for example by journal or name of first author. In my experience, many CD-ROM searches conducted by students fail to provide an adequate and specific set of references through lack of proper use of the features built into the software. In particular, learning to use the Index and Thesaurus properly can make your searches more sensitive and specific.

Obtaining access to research subjects

A wide range of approaches has been used by students in the past to carry out specific projects. Projects have been either qualitative or quantitative in approach, or have combined the two broad approaches to researching a question. Whatever method of approach is adopted, negotiating access to a particular group of research subjects or patients often requires considerable interpersonal skills and perseverance on the part of the researcher. You will be dependent upon the goodwill of people who will be helping you, and you do not have any right or authority to carry out research. Nevertheless, you can make the process easier for yourself if you stick to some ground rules. Thus a headteacher or administrator is unlikely to view sympathetically a request to use pupils or clients in a research study if the approach is made in such a way that they cannot be convinced of your integrety and the value of your research. If they are approached with a vague proposal, they may be unable to evaluate what you have in mind and give the safe answer, which is 'No'.

It is recommended that you make a formal written approach to the people concerned, outlining your ideas in some detail. If the outcome of the investigation may be of some benefit to the organisation or individuals, indicate that you will give them a copy of the findings. However, do not give the impression that the results may be of greater importance to the organisation than can reasonably be expected; remember that the outcome of many student projects is equivocal or inconclusive. You may need to negotiate a *quid pro quo*, so that, for instance, in a study concerned with the knowledge of schoolchildren about the benefits of exercise, you may offer to give talks to the classes on the subject, and incorporate this into your proposals.

Successful access to an organisation very often hinges on allaying sensitivities about the outcome and use of the research findings. Assurances of anonymity and confidentiality, so far as individuals in the study are concerned, may not be enough. You may also need to give undertakings that specific organisations or departments will not be mentioned in your report. It may be that you will need to modify the details of what you have in mind, if the alternative is to be refused access at all. However, before changing the overall approach of the project, remember that your particular study has been approved on your initial research proposal, and it is necessary that you at least discuss the nature of any proposed methodological changes with your supervisor.

Your research may be important to you but do not expect that people with whom you need to negotiate access will view it in the same light. People will sometimes put themselves out on your behalf in order to assist you without expecting anything in return, but the following extract from Judith Bell puts the point nicely.

> If at some time in the future, colleagues or other research workers ask you for your co-operation with a project, would you be willing to give the same amount of time and effort as you are asking for yourself? If not, perhaps you are asking too much.
>
> (Bell 1993:59)

Carrying out the study

Most students recognise that they need to pilot their methods before starting the main data collection. You may not have a great deal of time to conduct an extensive pilot study as a first step in data collection, but if you at least show a questionnaire to some colleagues and use perhaps five or ten people from your client group, you will detect any obvious errors and room for improvement on what you have developed. As discussed in Chapter 10, it is particularly important in studies which involve setting up interviews that you gain experience and confidence in conducting these through an initial pilot phase. In some qualitative projects, the piloting and main data collection may merge rather than being distinct phases. Laboratory methods, too, require piloting and developing of techniques before they are applied to collect data, and this phase may occupy a large proportion of the time available for a laboratory-based project.

Your project may be an action research one, that is, it is being carried out with practical aims in mind. Many other research studies in health come within the ambit of evaluations. Thus the effectiveness of procedures, policies or services may be subject to evaluation, including staff activities. The outcome of such studies may have potentially important consequences for the staff involved. There may be hostility to or suspicion of your methods or motives. Many students on health-related courses are also employed within the NHS or other organisations, and take the opportunity of carrying out their research projects in the workplace. You may need to overcome negative attitudes about the research by dint of tact, sensitivity and getting people on your side. You need to convince participants that you have high standards of integrity – no 'axe to grind' – in the study and are knowledgeable about the issues involved, including the political nuances.

Communication skills are an important dimension of successful research in real-life situations. Speaking with the right people, keeping people informed of what is proposed and what is going on can make all the difference to doors being opened for you in your research. If you can make it easy for people to take part in your research you are more likely to achieve co-operation. So a study designed to examine nursing activities on the ward is not likely to achieve a high degree of co-operation and acceptance if it requires hard pressed nursing staff regularly to fill in activity sheets. If people feel involved in the research process you are increasing your chances of gaining co-operation. They are unlikely to feel involved if a researcher breezes in to collect data and disappears afterwards, leaving little or no indication of the findings or conclusions. Providing feedback to those who have been involved is courteous, as are written expressions of thanks to participants.

Student research projects at undergraduate and postgraduate levels are always supervised and you should make full use of the supervision available to you. Do not be afraid to ask 'basic' questions or admit that things are not working out as planned. It is far better that your supervisor is aware of problems in good time to advise you about ways of overcoming them than that you carry on regardless in the hope that things will work out. Particularly critical stages where you should discuss things with your supervisor include the initial planning stage where decisions are made on the focus of the research question and the methods used to address the topic, and the stage of preparing to analyse the data. You may need to take advice from other people, such as a statistician, as well as your supervisor. Supervisors are there to help and advise you on the planning, conduct, analysis and reporting of your study, so establish a good relationship with your supervisor and see him or her regularly. Although procedures differ in different places, in general do not expect a supervisor to do the 'running around' for you; you will normally be responsible for obtaining permission, including ethics committee permission for your study, for arranging access to laboratories as appropriate and so on.

One of the secrets to conducting a successful piece of research is to adopt a methodical and organised approach to your activities. Appointments with research subjects should be kept in an appointments book, references should be organised in a filing system and laboratory experiments should be written up at the time in a lab notebook. If you document everything in this way, your task will be much easier when you come to write your project report. It is also helpful, especially in field projects extending over a period of months, to have a clear plan with a timetable so that you are sure of the sequence of stages through which you have to progress. Many activities in a project overlap and do not have distinct phases in practice, but normally certain tasks need to be accomplished before others and certain processes are 'critical' to the overall completion date, which is normally the date that a project report needs to be handed in. By identifying these activities, which may be the need to receive ethics committee approval by a certain date, the need to start collecting data by a certain date or the requirement to complete a questionnaire pilot at the same time as a sample is identified for the main study, the overall project will keep on track. In order to ensure that critical tasks are completed on time, to avoid delaying the overall project, you may need to devote extra time to them, shorten their duration if possible or start them earlier. One way of approaching this planning and organisation of a project is to draw up a Gantt chart. An example is shown in Figure 14.6 which lists 17 stages of a project concerned with evaluating the views of staff and patients at a health centre towards a reorganisation of services.

Although Figure 14.6 was produced using project management software, these charts can easily be drawn up manually if you do not have access to such a package. The chart clearly illustrates how non-critical tasks, such as the background literature searching, will not delay the project if they are not completed on time. The timing of most tasks, however, is critical, such as the need to to identify a sample and conduct a pilot study before the main study is conducted. If these slip they will delay the completion date for the outcome, which in this case is

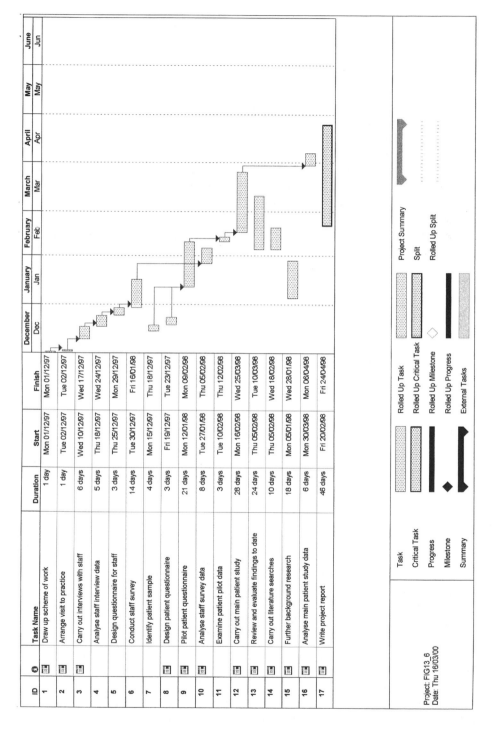

Figure 14.6 Gantt chart of stages involved in conducting a research study.

the latest date for the submission of a completed report on the project. In the Gantt chart, tasks which have to be done before others are started lie on the critical path and are indicated by linking arrows.

What if things go badly wrong?

The outcomes of the research study may be as you had hoped when it was conceived. For all sorts of reasons, however, in practice things can and do go wrong. For example, in a laboratory-based study, it is by no means uncommon for a published method simply to refuse to work under your conditions. The bulk of your project time may then be spent in modifications to get an experiment working instead of collecting data on the original problem. This is a risk with any research study at any level; the experience can generate anxiety in a 'results-driven' culture or when examiners are assessing the outcomes of a project. The chances are that the examiners, if they are at all well experienced in research, will have been in a comparable position in their research careers and will be concerned with how you tackle the problems encountered. There is no need to regard a project as a 'failure' simply because things did not work out as you had hoped. Do not be despondent; the position could be salvaged. Comments on the process can often be as insightful as any hard conclusions about outcomes might have been. Of this, Pat Cryer in her excellent volume aimed at the postgraduate student writes:

> ... the research student may be able to capitalize on everything that goes wrong. Important equipment may not work; critical resources may not be available; people may not agree to be interviewed; funding may be withdrawn; or there may be other serious and unforseen obstacles ... a little creative thinking can rescue the situation. There are almost always byproducts during any research, perhaps the development of a certain piece of equipment or some interesting secondary findings in the literature. These can be moved into the mainstream of the research, and focused on or developed further. ... the research problem merely needs to be reformulated to reflect the new nature of the work.
>
> (Cryer 1996:148)

You may need to allow a period of some weeks after data collection finishes to complete the writing of your project report. Tackling this is the topic of the next chapter.

Action points

- Continue to build up your collection of relevant literature.
- Read relevant books on the methodology you have chosen.
- Negotiate all access required at the appropriate stages.
- Plan out the organisation and conduct of the study.
- Conduct and evaluate the results of a pilot study.
- Carry out the main data collection.
- Document everything as you go along.

Chapter 15

Writing your project report

Writing your project report should help to crystallise your thinking about the research which you have carried out. As one author, Ian Dey, has written:

> What you cannot explain to others, you do not understand yourself. Producing an account of our analysis is not just something we do for an audience. It is also something we do for ourselves. Producing an account is not just a question of reporting results; it is also another method of producing these results. Through the challenge of explaining ourselves to others, we can help to clarify and integrate concepts and relationships we have identified in our analysis.

(Dey 1993:00)

It is not advisable to leave all your writing up to the last minute after you have collected your data. Your literature review and introduction may be written, at least in draft form, at an early stage during the execution of your project. The methods section too does not usually significantly alter after you have completed your pilot study, although you may wish to delay writing the description of the statistical tests you have used until the analysis is complete. Your database of relevant literature, much of which you will have located early on in the project, will be added to as the research unfolds. I have suggested elsewhere that you organise your references using a database or card index system. Normally, the last major section to be written is the discussion, once you have thought about the implications of the findings in considerable detail.

Your project report should conform to the conventions of journal report writing and should not use personal pronouns, should be written in the past tense and should be fully and appropriately referenced. It needs to be said that some authorities on the writing up of qualitative research would not necessarily agree with this objective approach and would claim that first person narrative can sometimes offer an advantage. The general point is that you would not state that 'Jane and I carried out a study in Chichester' but would restate this as 'A study was carried out in Chichester by two researchers'.

A principal characteristic of scientific writing is that it is precise. Many statements that pass by without a blink in the course of normal conversation would be out of place in a scientific report because they are open to a variety of interpretations, or are value loaded. Words like 'moderate', 'overwhelming' and 'several' may mean different things to different people and researchers try to avoid ambiguity in their writing. Words like 'outrageous', 'wonderful' or 'pathetic' are also generally out of place in a research report since they are highly value loaded and may tell us much about the values and attitudes of the author but do not necessarily add to our understanding of the research.

It has been claimed that scientific writing is standardised, homogenised and boring because it has to meet the criteria outlined above. Whilst the principal purpose of a research report is essentially to communicate, the writing need not be dry and pedantic; by reading some of the best research papers and books by scientific writers you can learn to acquire the skills of making your research communications factual and insightful as well as interesting to read. Great care should be taken over the presentation of your final report. A well laid out and presented report, free of typographical errors, with charts and tables clearly and accurately labelled will immediately create a favourable impression or 'aura' in the mind of those reading it concerning the care that you have taken. This positive psychological set can influence their attitude towards your whole report.

It is widespread policy to encourage the use of non-sexist language and non-discriminatory language in general. Research subjects including people of both genders should preferably be referred to therefore as 's/he' rather than the traditional 'he'. Your phrasing can usually be recast to avoid gender specific references when these are not accurate or appropriate. 'Man has for centuries …' can become more accurately 'People have for centuries ...'. If you refer to people chairing a committee in general (rather than a specific committee which you know is chaired by a male), it should accurately be 'the chairperson' or 'chair' rather than 'the chairman'. Our language has in all sorts of ways been used a powerful means of reinforcing outdated stereotypes. The guidelines on anti-sexist language produced by the British Sociological Association also ask researchers to consider the extent to which their work may be heterosexist; for example, in discussions about women and sexuality, is it being assumed that 'sexually active' means becoming sexually active with men?

The overall scheme of a research report is usually along the following lines:

- Title
- Summary (or abstract)
- Introduction or background
- Methodology
- Results or findings
- Discussion/Conclusions
- References
- Appendices if appropriate.

The title

The title should be short and descriptive of the study. You are pointing a reader to the main theme of the investigation and nothing more. Examples of concise yet informative titles from papers appearing in medical literature are shown below:

- Is general practitioner decision making associated with patient socio-economic status?
- Food choice: a conceptual model of the process
- Associations between drug use and deviant behaviour in teenagers
- Does the human visual system implement an ideal observer theory of slant from texture?
- Social networks, social support and coping with serious illness: the family connection
- Involvement of nitric oxide in nitroprusside-induced hepatocyte cytotoxicity
- Anxiety sensitivity: confirmatory evidence for a multidimensional construct.

If the research report is being prepared as a paper for publication, some potential readers will search on key words appearing in the title. Note from the above list that the topic of the investigations is clear in each case and some are clearly exploratory studies, others correlational in nature and others experimental.

The abstract or summary

The summary is normally the last part of a research report to be written. It should provide a balanced overview, normally in a few hundred words, of the main aims, methods, findings and conclusions of the research. The summary is the only part of a research report or paper that many readers will attend to; if it is part of a paper submitted for publication it will be made available to a much wider audience, through databases such as MEDLINE and Psychological Abstracts, than the full paper will ever reach.

The following is an abstract of a research paper entitled 'Do the homeless get a fair deal from general practitioners?'

Many studies have indicated the health status of homeless people to be typically poorer than that of the general population, with various studies indicating a high prevalence of psychiatric illness, drug or alcohol misuse and associated socio-medical problems. The Bristol Primary Healthcare Project is an agency which was established to provide a local health care service tailored to the needs of people who are homeless. The present study was carried out as part of an evaluation of the service offered locally to homeless people by general practitioners. A postal questionnaire survey of 155 general practices within the Avon FHSA area was carried out. Both fundholding and non-fundholding practices were included, within an area including inner city, urban and rural/semi-rural locations. One hundred and seventeen completed questionnaires were returned, providing a response rate of 75%. Twenty-seven percent of practices would fully register a homeless person who seeks to register at the practice, 24% would treat as immediate and necessary and 33% would treat as a temporary resident. Four percent of fundholding practices surveyed would fully register homeless persons and 55% of inner city practices would do so. Seventy-nine percent of doctors indicated that homeless patients were more difficult to treat than other patients. The most frequent problems associated with registering homeless people were perceived to be the associated social problems (90% of respondents agreed), the lack of medical records (88% agreed), the complex health problems (79% agreed) and the associated alcohol or substance misuse (78% agreed). The study has highlighted a need for government to consider providing incentives to general practitioners to register homeless people without resulting in adverse effects on their contract targets. The reluctance of some practices to register these patients varied by area and type of practice with doctors at fundholding practices being the most reluctant. There is an identified need for further health education and promotion work and initiatives exemplified by the Bristol Primary Health Care Project for people who are homeless.

(Wood, Wilkinson and Kumar, 1997)

Many journals specify that an abstract is written in a particular way, known as a structured abstract. The headings of a typical structured abstract would be:

- Objective
- Design
- Setting
- Participants
- Main outcome measures
- Conclusions.

Even if your research report does not specify a structured abstract, it can be good practice to adopt this scheme, to make sure that the salient features of the study are presented in a logical way in the summary. Not all studies, however, particularly qualitative reports, will necessarily fit in neatly with the above scheme.

The introduction

The introduction to a research report should have a logical structure to it. A common approach is to start with a literature review citing papers of importance to the area of inquiry and bringing in theoretical issues and their connections as the introduction unfolds. The literature reviewed may start off with general papers around the topic of interest, then subsequently focus on directly relevant work as the review unfolds. Do not report studies which are not of relevance to your investigation, simply because you have unearthed them and wish to bulk out your list of references; this will weaken a report. The major findings or conclusions should be stated in a literature review, not the methodological details. In a literature review, you will be expected to adopt a critical and analytical approach to the work reviewed; a literature review which simply repeats lists of findings and conclusions will not meet this criterion. However, you should have an evidence base for specific criticisms of reports and papers; this evidence base comes from other papers you should have read.

The introduction normally proceeds to describe the study actually carried out. It may end with the stating of a research hypothesis. Not all studies have to have one or more hypotheses, however; many studies carried out are exploratory in nature, such as cross-sectional surveys, and it is not essential to state hypotheses for these in the introductory section of your report. All studies, however, have one or more aims and objectives in conducting the research and these should be clearly stated in the introduction. In qualitative studies, where the initial aims may be relatively unfocused and proceed as the research unfolds, it is important to be clear about the aims and purposes of the research and these should be stated in your introduction. If your research has a particular hypothesis, this should be clearly and succinctly stated; this may revolve around the predicted relationship of one or more independent variables upon the dependent variable. The formal approach is to state the null hypothesis along with the research hypothesis, although this practice is becoming less common.

Note how the points mentioned above have been taken into account in the introduction to the Wood, Wilkinson and Kumar (1997) paper.

> Some 1–2 million people may be homeless in the UK at any one time, depending upon how this is defined, and estimates have been made that there may be 20,000 individuals who sleep rough from time to time (Shelter 1991). There are many groups falling within the ambit of the homeless label including New Age travellers, hostel dwellers discharged from long stay psychiatric institutions and the temporarily homeless. Surveys have indicated that most homeless people are men, but that about 10–25 per cent are

women, of whom about half are accompanied by children (Scott 1993). Comparatively little is known of the social and medical characteristics of people who sleep rough although initiatives have included the provision of mobile surgeries to provide primary health care in central London where many homeless people sleep outdoors (Ransden *et al.* 1989). Findings indicate the patients are seen to be generally a group with deprived and unstable backgrounds, sometimes compounded by alcohol misuse. A study of factors associated with street injecting of polydrug users showed a high level of severe drug dependence together with associated health problems and a high proportion were homeless (Klee and Morris 1995).

A census carried out in Sheffield in 1991 (George *et al.* 1991) aimed to examine social and medical characteristics of single homeless people. Various chronic medical conditions were reported and the perceived health status of the population was low with a high prevalence of psychiatric illness. Most of the group studied obtained health care from general practitioners, but less than two-thirds were registered with a GP. A further study in Sheffield using the SF-36 health status instrument amongst a sample of hostel residents found high levels of health service use and poor average perceived health by comparison with other groups in the population (Usherwood and Jones 1993). The health status of the temporarily homeless of North West Thames was examined by a study reported in 1992 (Victor, 1992). Although the rates of acute illness amongst this group were similar to those reported by regional residents, as was the prevalence of long-standing illness, the prevalence of mental morbidity was twice that of residents in the region as a whole. The prevalence of mental disorder in residents of hostels for the homeless in Belfast was explored using interviews with officers in charge (McAuley and McKenna 1995). That study indicated that about one-quarter of that group had a diagnosed mental disorder and further it was concluded that hospital closures had had an impact on this figure. Support from the health service was found to be unsatisfactory.

At least one other study (Marshall and Reed 1992) has indicated the prevalence of schizophrenia in a group of homeless women from hostels in inner London to be as high as 64 per cent. It has been argued that the reported psychiatric morbidity of many homeless persons may be a direct result of their homelessness and poverty and further that the rates of psychiatric morbidity amongst the homeless may have been overestimated as a result of sampling problems (Abdul Hamid *et al.* 1993). In a study in central London of homeless staying in bed and breakfast accommodation and sleeping rough who had contacted statutory or voluntary agencies in the area, the prevalence of psychiatric problems was found to vary greatly with age and gender (Fisher *et al*, 1994).

A survey of 2000 homeless people applying for shelter to statutory and voluntary sector agencies in Nottingham (Whynes and Giggs 1992) examined the incidence of reported health indicators in this group with data from the 1988 General Household Survey (GHS). It was found that although overall they were a young and relatively healthy sample, particular groups of the homeless exhibited a disproportionate amount of ill health compared to the GHS population. In recent years there has been growing concern that tuberculosis may be spreading in Europe in the way that it is in the USA (Kent 1993). Using a DNA fingerprinting technique to uncover foci of transmission the largest groups included drug users, homeless persons and alcoholics (Genewein *et al*, 1993) and there appeared to be a spillover to the general population. Furthermore, multi-drug resistant tuberculosis developed in this setting. At least one study (Stevens *et al.* 1992) has concluded that mass miniature X-ray screening is ineffective in controlling tuberculosis in a group of single homeless hostel residents as a result of its unacceptability and the increased inaccessibility to this population. It has been concluded that the national rise in tuberculosis affects only the poorest areas in the UK (Bhatti *et al*. 1995) and further that pathways associated with HIV transmission are associated with poverty and have a relationship to factors including homelessness (Gillies *et al*. 1996)

There is therefore recent research describing some of the health problems and socio-medical characteristics of groups of homeless people. However, the evaluation of potential service solutions has received relatively little attention. It has been stated that primary care for the homeless in the UK lacks central government direction, suffers from an overlap of statutory agencies and is disproportionately delivered in emergency rooms (Reuler 1989). This comparative lack of NHS provision increases the marginalisation of the homeless. One initiative is the Bristol Primary Healthcare Project which was established to provide health care services tailored to meet the needs of people who are homeless in Bristol. Initial funding was provided by the Department of Health in 1992. In addition to the core services provided by the Project Team, that is doctors and nurses, the nurses undertake regular outreach sessions both with Bristol Cyrenians and Avon Council on Alcohol and Drugs (Heavy Street Drinkers Initiative) and also a weekly psychiatric session is being provided by a consultant psychiatrist.

The programme of the Bristol Primary Health Care Project for people who are homeless includes an emphasis on health education and promotion work with young people. This work includes helping young homeless people to design and produce posters and leaflets for example around drug-related issues and TB and taking part in group discussions. Members of the team have been working with a Consultant in Communicable Diseases Control in Bristol in respect of the prevalence of tuberculosis amongst homeless people in the City. The Project Team provide clinical sessions at a day centre and a hostel and the core team consists of three doctors working part time, two full-time nurses and a part-time receptionist/secretary with additional clerical and administrative support. As part of this overall initiative a survey was undertaken to determine the views of general practitioners within the Avon area in order to determine their perceptions of the difficulties of dealing with homeless people and practice policies towards the registration of this group of people.

(Wood, Wilkinson and Kumar 1997)

The methodology

The methods section of a paper or research report is normally composed of a number of different sections. The methods section should convey clearly and unambiguously exactly what was carried out in the study, whether it was an observational study or an experimental one. Your aim here should be to provide the reader with sufficient information to repeat the study and emerge with the same or essentially similar findings. This is called replication of a study and is an important part of the evaluation of the worth of scientific findings. The design of the study should be set out in the methods section. This may be fairly brief if it is a cross-sectional survey. If the study was experimental in nature, you need to state whether it was a between-subjects (independent groups) or repeated measures (within subjects) design or alternatively matched groups design. You also need to state what the independent and dependent variables were.

Another section of the methodology frequently contains a description of the participants or subjects of the study. You are expected to specify the important characteristics of the subjects involved. That is, they may be volunteers or may have been selected according to certain characteristics, such as being between certain ages and so on. Inclusion criteria and exclusion criteria need to be stated. If certain characteristics of subjects or patients were required, such as the presence of certain symptoms, these need to be stated along with the method of decision and selection based upon these criteria. Many studies use student volunteers or people stopped in the street. (The limitations of these samples need to be recognised and addressed, although this would not be done in the methodology. Any factors which could affect the generalisability of the study would be considered in the discussion section of your report.)

Any materials and apparatus used in a study should also be described in the methodology section. The precise make and model, and particular settings such as the sensitivity setting of pen recorders, the number of channels used and so on are all likely to be important information and should be included. The final sub-heading of a methods section normally describes the procedure which was carried out. This is a factual and chronological description of the course of events in the study. The methods section from a paper by Turnbull, Wood and Kester (1998) entitled 'Controlled trial of the subjective benefits of walking to the operating theatre' is divided into two short sections as follows:

Participants

One hundred surgical patients attending a private hospital in the South of England were included in the trial. All were consecutive patients meeting the entry criteria and chosen over a six week period in 1996 from a short-stay mixed-sex and mixed-speciality ward catering for general, orthopaedic, ENT, gynaecological and ophthalmic surgery. Excluded from the trial were patients requiring pre-medication, those aged under 18 years, those undergoing intra-ocular surgery and any whom the medical staff judged to be too ill, too infirm or whose mobility was too impaired to take part. All eligible patients were randomised either to an experimental (walking) or control (trolley) group. A pilot study involved 10 patients selected on the same criteria as above.

Procedure

Hospital ethical committee clearance was obtained, also permission from each consultant associated associated with the hospital. Before their operation, all participants were given a short questionnaire which they were asked to complete and return to the field researcher (a member of hospital nursing staff) prior to their discharge. Informed consent was obtained from each participant who read and signed an information sheet explaining the background and purpose of the study. The questionnaires contained items concerning:

- basic demographic information
- previous experience of surgery
- pre-operative anxiety and concerns
- choice concerning method of conveyance to theatre
- perceived quality of care
- free text comments (optional).

All data from these questionnaires were coded and entered onto a database. Data generated from the numeric items were from nominal scales and frequency counts and cross-tabulation using the chi-square test and the Fisher exact test, for 2×2 tables with small expected frequencies, were applied using the SPSS package.

(Turnbull, Wood and Kester 1998)

The results

The findings of a study are reported here, without any interpretation or discussion of their implications, which is reserved for the final (discussion) section of a paper or report. The data generated may be qualitative or quantitative. If quantitative data has been generated, the results should be presented in the most appropriate ways. These may include written description of the findings, tables, charts and diagrams. If qualitative data has been obtained it is often a good idea to summarise the categories which have emerged from a qualitative analysis as a tree diagram, as is shown in Figure 10.2, together with exemplars of text within each category that have been chosen to support the category.

Descriptive statistics summarise the properties of data, that is, they present measures of average and measures of variation in the data. A table of standard deviations and means is informative for data which has been measured at an interval or ratio level, whereas a table of medians is appropriate if the data comprises measurements from ordinal scales. You should generally not include much raw data in the results section: it may appear in an appendix to a research report, whereas the results should summarise the findings in a digestible form. The results of the application of inferential statistics are normally also required for quantitative data; these, for example, report the significance of associations between variables using correlation coefficients or differences between groups using Mann–Whitney or independent or paired t tests or analysis of variance, depending upon the level of measurement and the design of the study, as discussed in Chapter 8. You only need to mention the type of test used, the value of the obtained statistic, the degrees of freedom associated with the sample size used and the probability level. The probability level quoted should not be the exact probability level obtained on a printout; this should be rounded to the nearest preferred value, such as $p < 0.05$, $p < 0.001$ and so forth.

Any tables which appear in the results should have a table number and a caption. The caption should be a piece of explanatory text indicating what the table is presenting. Similarly, any charts that you include should be clearly labelled with a key to the bars or lines used and include a figure number which can be referred to in the text.

The discussion

The results section of a report simply states what the findings were. However, a reader will also need to know what caused an association or a difference, which may not have been related to the investigation at all. There may be confounding variables which could account for the result, at least in principle. We need to decide between the various explanations for a result and to recognise any limitations on the interpretation of the findings. We also need to relate the findings to the existing literature. All of these tasks are accomplished in the discussion section of a paper. Like other sections, a discussion should be logically structured and arranged.

A discussion frequently starts off by re-introducing the main findings in a wider context of interpretation and discussion of their meaning. The next part of the discussion frequently addresses limitations of the study. If a researcher cannot assess the limitations of a study it is a sure bet that others will, and if these are not addressed in the discussion by the author, a reader may draw the conclusion that you have not been able to recognise them. On the other hand, there is no need to be too self-critical; every study has its own limitations and the important thing is to recognise when there may be genuine weaknesses in the study which may limit the conclusions, such as the appropriateness of the sample or the design. The findings of many studies tend to be over-generalised, whereas there are usually limitations imposed by geography, the sample, the methods of control used, the validity of the questionnaire and so on, which all need to be recognised and taken account of in the discussion of the outcome of a particular study.

It is frequent practice to conclude the discussion of a study by pointing to further research which may be required to answer remaining questions, or new questions thrown up by the study. This may be further research which you are intending to carry out and this is the place to sketch out the proposed path of the research if it is a logical extension of the work that you have just reported. Studies where the results are inconsistent with other findings in the field need especially careful interpretation. However, if you are confident that the study has been carried out well, there is no need to assume that your results are aberrant; there may be an explanation which is based upon a particular design feature of your study or the type of sample employed, and your findings may well help illuminate, or even question, other findings in the field.

The discussion section from the Wood, Wilkinson and Kumar paper is included next, so that you can see how it was structured in the light of the comments above.

> This study has revealed a great deal about the attitudes and perceptions of G.P.s towards homeless people. Although any local study of the views of general practitioners can be criticised on the grounds that it is not fully representative of general practitioners throughout the UK, the geographical spread of practices included in the survey included affluent rural/semi-rural and suburban areas as well as deprived inner city areas in Bristol. Replies were received from three-quarters of practices surveyed and we have no reason to assume that the responses were not typical of practices across a range of settings.
>
> Full registration of patients implies an obligation to visit and follow up patients which was regarded as a difficult task with some homeless people. Some G.P.s mentioned the effects on contract targets such as immunisation targets and Table 2 indicates that 60 per cent expressed this as a concern. The evidence of this survey indicates that there may be a need for central initiative to consider providing an incentive for a greater number of G.P.s to register homeless people without adverse effects on contract targets. It is pertinent to note that a much higher percentage of practices located within inner city areas (56 per cent) would fully register homeless people and the homeless are more likely to present in these districts. Familiarity and experience of dealing with homeless people may lead to a greater acceptance on the part of the practices involved and comments were received from partners at a number of practices indicating that such patients were sometimes perceived as unwelcome, troublesome, dirty, smelly and off-putting to other patients in the waiting room. New Age travellers were frequently mentioned in this respect in freely volunteered comments received from individual G.P.s. It can be noted that a study examining factors influencing response to advertisements for general practice vacancies indicated a greater difficulty in recruiting general practitioners in areas

with the highest proportion of patients eligible for deprivation payments (Carlisle and Johnstone 1996) and consequently the greatest health needs.

It is pertinent to note that significantly fewer inner city practices agreed that there was a difficulty in referring such patients to secondary care services, again probably reflecting greater experience gained in practice. It can be noted in this respect that a prospective case control study of admissions in a London hospital indicated that referrals of homeless children for acute medical admissions were made by a general practitioner in only 10 per cent of the homeless compared to 36 per cent of controls (Lissauer *et al.* 1993).

About 8 out of 10 practices perceived the homeless as more difficult to treat than the average patient and the most frequently cited form of additional support the G.P.s would welcome was the provision of a Homeless Advice Centre. Additional information on local support groups was also welcomed by over half the practices surveyed. By contrast the problem was not perceived as one requiring additional resources by the majority of practices, nor was additional training of G.P.s perceived as a widespread need.

A prevailing ethos of the National Health Service is equity of care and access to services depending upon need and not social or financial factors. It is clear, from the evidence of this survey and from much other evidence, that homeless people, especially those living rough with no fixed abode, are in many cases falling through the net of care. The problem is not confined to the provision of GP services. For example a study in Leeds indicated that there was a high level of normative need for dental care amongst single male hostel dwellers, despite a low level of expressed need (Blackmore *et al.* 1995).

Whilst the reasons for the lack of provision for the homeless are complex and varied one factor is the reluctance of some practices to wish to treat these people. Comments were received from individual G.P.s who regarded these groups as being particularly demanding and manipulative and there was a frequently mentioned difficulty of the need to provide continuity of care for patients who move around and that referrals could be difficult without a contact number or address. Some FHSAs may be unwilling to accept no fixed abode as an address on their records and policy may need to be re-examined. Whilst the provision of mobile surgeries and temporary emergency treatment can be helpful, the policy of some practices may need to be re-examined. It is noteworthy for example that of 24 fundholding practices included in this study, only one would fully register homeless people (Table 1). We have no evidence concerning how typical this finding may be of fundholding practices in general in the UK, but potentially fundholding practices, especially concerned about meeting contract targets, have little incentive to register patients in this category. When the fundholding scheme was first put forward fears were raised that practices might be tempted to 'cream skim' (Weiner and Ferris 1990) although the results of early evaluation provided no evidence to bear this out (Glennerster *et al.* 1992). The evidence of this study indicates that complacency in this respect should not prevail. The recently elected Labour government have pledged to end the internal market as it presently exists and that GPs and nurses will be expected to take a lead in planning local health services for all the patients in their area (Labour Party Manifesto, 1997).

In respect of the data collected in the survey reported here, data from this reporting period indicated that 33 per cent (128) of clients who used the Project for the first time were registered with a general practitioner in Avon and 59 per cent were not registered either in Avon or with a GP elsewhere. In respect of registered patients, the Jarman index is used to calculate the allowance that general practices receive for each registered patient who lives in an area of social deprivation, although this process has been criticised as a result of under counting of homeless people (Majeed *et al.* 1996).

The registration procedure and record keeping have been seen as major obstacles preventing homeless people receiving appropriate primary health care services. If a person wishing to register with a GP does not have a fixed address they may be able to provide an accommodation address which may be that of a friend, a day centre or even the FHSA or the GPs surgery. In ways such as this, it is desirable to encourage practices to register homeless people as permanent rather than temporary residents in order to improve the continuity of their care.

(Wood, Wilkinson and Kumar 1997)

Referencing your report

In articles which appear in scientific journals, a list of all papers and books which have been cited in the text is required. There are a number of alternative ways of including references in papers or in your report, and each journal specifies this in the 'Instructions for authors' section. It is a common enough mistake to cite an author's work in the text of the report but fail to list the reference at the end of a report. It is not a case of 'the more you cite the better' – the number invariably depends on the topic you have chosen, the amount of previous work carried out and so on. However, the general rule is that, if you make a statement which is not either common knowledge or would be expected to be agreed by a reader in the area you are discussing, the statement should be backed up by a reference to a published piece of work. The most typical sections to cite references would be in the introduction and in the discussion but you may also wish to reference statements made in the methods and findings sections.

Authors referred to can be included in the project report in a number of ways. Sometimes a system of using consecutive numbers is adopted to reference statements made. The alternative is to provide authors' names and year of publication in the text. For example:

Wood (1989) reported that ...

Kester (1995) stated that ...

According to Platzer (1997) it has ...

It has been shown (Rose *et al.* 1981) ...

A study undertaken by Muir-Gray (1999) suggests ...

You will find it helpful to develop a repertoire of standard phrases that will help you incorporate references into your writing. As you read, make a note of other useful phrases that you encounter. Where a paper has been written by more than two co-authors, give the name of the first author in your report and refer to the rest as '*et al.*' ('and others') as in the Rose *et al.* example shown above. In your list of references at the end of your report, you would give the names of all the authors of the Rose *et al.* paper.

If you have been told something verbally or in a letter by a person with knowledge or authority and you wish to use this information in your report, the convention is to refer to this in the text of your report as follows:

> According to Professor Pam Smith (personal communication, 1999) the effect of …

When quoting directly from an author you should include quotation marks, the author's name and date of publication, and the page number. For example:

> According to Stephenson, 'Registered nurses who become students in higher educational institutes often require some assistance in reaching the "right" level of content in their academic essays' (Stephenson 1985:120)

In the list of references appearing at the end of your report, all of the authors who have been cited would appear as a list arranged alphabetically by surname.

You will need to be especially vigilant when using books that are edited by one or more people and have chapters written by a number of subject experts. In this case you should include the reference at the end of your project report as follows:

> Clarke, E. (1989) 'Hybrid courses in continuing professional development', in Robinson, K.M. (ed) (1989) *Open and Distance Learning for Nurses*, Longman.

Sometimes you will not be able to consult a primary source yourself, but will have to read about it in someone else's work. In this case you are using a secondary source, and it must be acknowledged as such. For example, if you read about Piaget's work on cognitive development in a psychology textbook, you would refer to it in your report in the following way:

> In 1953, Piaget studied... (cited in Atkison *et al*. 1987)

Then, in the listing of your references you would put Piaget alphabetically and then add 'cited in …' as follows:

> Piaget, J. (1953) *The Origins of Intelligence in Children*, New York: International Universities Press, cited in Atkinson, R.L., Atkinson, R.C., Smith, E.E. and Hilgard, E.R. (1987) *Introduction to Psychology* (9th edn), Harcourt Brace Jovanovitch.

Appendices

Appendices should contain all information you have collected relevant to your study, such as the results of statistical analyses in printouts, the raw data, letters of permission obtained from subjects or managers, sample questionnaires used, full transcripts of interviews for qualitative studies and so on. Appendices enable you to expand on the information included in your write-up of the study and are a source of reference for those reading the report, should a particular detail wish to be checked. It needs to be said, however, that appendices are sometimes not read by readers of a report, or by its markers, and therefore anything which is essential to understanding what you have done should not be included in an appendix but should appear in the main body of the text as appropriate. Do not therefore present a sketch of the findings in the results section and leave all the detailed charts in an appendix; they should be included in the main report.

The above structure for a report or paper may not fit in well with the conduct and analysis of some qualitative studies. For example, in the results section in a study which has involved the analysis of interview transcripts, you may feel it necessary to include a great deal of theory generation and interpretation.

When your project is finally complete and written up, or at some stage afterwards, you may need to present your results verbally at class presentations, seminars and so forth. Some things to keep in mind when doing this are discussed in the next chapter.

Action points

- Decide on the overall framework of material that you will include.
- Write the introduction and literature review at an early stage.
- Document and write up your methods at the time.
- As soon as analysis is finished, complete the writing of your draft.
- Read and check your drafts carefully.
- Submit a finished report by the due date.

Chapter 16

Telling it like it was ...

It is normal practice for researchers to communicate verbally and present their results to peer groups. Thus professional researchers give seminars, present their results at conferences and so forth. This is an important part of assisting the process of dissemination of research findings as well as gaining feedback on the reactions of other researchers and experts in the field in which you are working.

When giving a project presentation, or indeed any verbal communication to an audience, you will need to prepare your material beforehand. It is not advisable simply to write down exactly what you are going to say and read it verbatim; although this may give you more confidence, it is much less engaging for the listeners than a more interactive talk. Instead, you can adopt a number of alternative methods of presenting your work. In your presentation, you can prepare overhead projector (OHP) slides which provide 'bullet points' to structure your talk; the first few slides may refer to key papers and their findings, the next one or two to methodological points, followed by some tables or charts to present your summary results and a concluding slide listing your key conclusions. That way, you have a structure to cue you as to what to say next, without every word being written out beforehand. The software package Powerpoint, or other presentation software, enables professional-looking overhead slides to be prepared easily with a PC and an ink-jet printer. Special transparencies can be bought which enable colour slides to be produced on a standard ink-jet printer; the expense is worthwhile for a special presentation. Figures 16.1 and 16.2 provide examples of Powerpoint slides; the former illustrates a bulleted methods slide and the latter a results slide.

A standard word processor, however, can also give good results. Remember the golden rules: do not put too much information on any one slide (a dozen or so lines is generally the most that should be attempted), and keep the text font large (at least 18 point is recommended, so people at the back of the room can see clearly).

Novice speakers may find that practising the presentation at home and listening to it on a tape recording can give them further confidence. For an important presentation, perhaps one which is part of a formal assessment, you may consider having a practice run-through in front of some friends who can give you honest feedback on your manner and style. Some speakers find that they like to have a list of key points written on index cards, even if they use OHP slides.

Giving a project presentation can be an anxious experience for many. Remember that you are the expert on your own piece of research and will undoubtedly be more familiar with the specific literature and work you have carried out than anyone else in the room. A polished and lucid presentation of your results, using OHP and other material as appropriate, will create a favourable impression. A clear and coherent presentation can help the listeners in

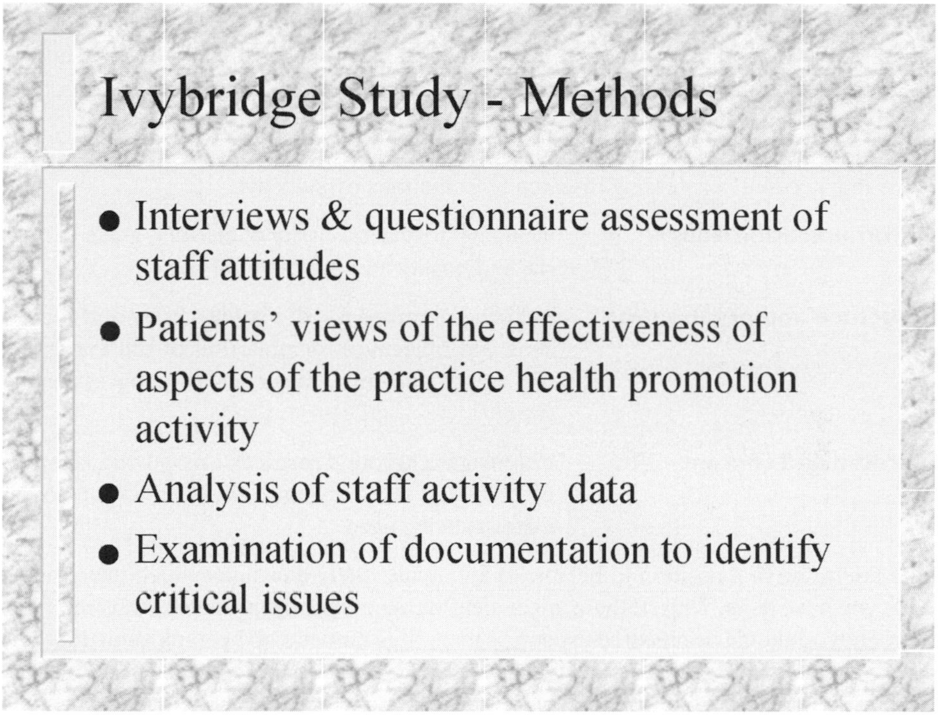

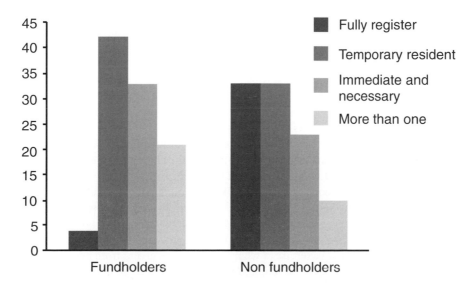

Figure 16.1 Microsoft Powerpoint slide: bullet list of methods.

Figure 16.2 Microsoft Powerpoint slide: results.

understanding a piece of work. On the other hand, a rambling and ill thought out presentation is not likely to add any new insights into what you have done. Preparation of handouts for the audience to summarise the key points of your presentation is very often a good idea. If you have used presentation software such as 'Powerpoint' to prepare your slides, handouts can easily be printed in various styles such as a sheet of screenprints of your slides, together with space for audience notes.

At the School of Health at University College Chichester, the following points have been taken into account in assessing research presentations by students.

Communication skills	including originality, clarity of delivery, grasp of material and quality and use of visual aids
Structure and organisation	including rationale for the study, clarity and focus of aims and objectives, organisation of the material to the target audience, sequence of progression and variety
Material and content	including background research carried out, relevance of material, accuracy and evidence of up-to-date material being used

You are in the best position to be able to anticipate likely questions which may arise about what you have done. Thus, if there are evident weaknesses or gaps in your research (which is normal), you should be prepared to address them. It is far better to be frank about these than to attempt to claim more for the study than is deserved. Flaws in the study can be addressed constructively in relation to lessons that have been learned in practice about the design or specific methods which were used. To attempt to minimise their impact, or even to conceal them, is likely to be counterproductive since they may be obvious to others in the room with more experience of research. On the other hand, some student research presentations are almost apologetic in their approach, and this displays a lack of confidence in what has been done. Even if the study was inconclusive or suffered major setbacks in practice, most studies have their redeeming features and will be of interest if honestly and unpretentiously presented. Telling the story of your research project as it happened, warts and all, is an honest approach which is likely to gain empathy from the audience. It is a good idea to have on hand some spare slides which you have prepared which may be shown to help you respond to questions which may arise in the discussion.

The interpretation of the evidence from a research study, whatever method of data collection and analysis has been used, is always open to challenge and negotiation between observers. Consider the example mentioned in Chapter 3, concerning the survey which has shown a link between poor health status and unemployment. If the alternative interpretations that 'unemployment is detrimental to your health' and that 'poor health status tends to lead to unemployment' were not both considered in the light of all the data which was obtained, the researcher might find his/her interpretations challenged. Whilst in a written communication you are not likely to receive this feedback in any immediate way, it might well happen in a verbal presentation. An oral communication of your methods, findings and interpretations is therefore a valuable learning exercise at whatever level it is given, from peer scrutiny at class presentations to peer scrutiny of communications given at national and international conferences.

Action points

- Carefully prepare your material for the presentation, taking into account the intended audience.
- Do not cram your visual aids with too much information and make sure they are clearly readable from a distance.
- Practise your presentation at home or in front of some friends if you need further confidence.

Chapter 17

Putting together a critical analysis

Very often in research methods courses, especially at diploma rather than final year degree level, you are not required to carry out a piece of research involving the collection of new data. Instead, you may may be asked to analyse critically a piece of research in published form. This chapter is intended to provide some guidelines for this process. Providing a critical analysis of a research paper should draw upon all the skills and knowledge of the research process that I have aimed to impart throughout this volume.

You may be given a research paper, or group of related papers, to criticise. More commonly, you are asked to choose a research study yourself. The first piece of advice, therefore, is to choose your research paper carefully. Make sure it is something that will retain your interest throughout the hours of background research required to put together a proper critical analysis. Most importantly, choose one in a field you know something about, either because of professional involvement or because you have read around the topic. Choose a paper, or papers, that provide substantial details of the research study in a recognised academic or professional journal; it is not usually appropriate to attempt a critical analysis of a popular summary of a study published in magazines such as the *Health Services Journal*.

In approaching your critical analysis, amongst the first questions you may wish to consider are:

- Who conducted the research?
- Where was it carried out?
- Where was it published?
- Who funded the research?

Thus the authors' credentials should be borne in mind: are their qualifications and experience appropriate to the topic being researched? Was the study carried out in the UK or the USA or somewhere else, and is this relevant to professional practice? There is a huge variety of research journals that publish health-related material and they vary in quality, especially in the processes or standards of peer review that are applied to articles submitted for publication by researchers. The better known and international journals – such as the *British Medical Journal*, the *Journal of Advanced Nursing* or the *Journal of the American Medical Association* to name but a few – generally apply rigorous standards of review of articles submitted. Do not automatically assume, however, that because a research paper appears in a prestigious journal that it is necessarily true or beyond reproach. Also consider who it was that funded the study; funding organisations range from charities, research councils and local sources to commercial companies such as drug and appliance manufacturers. Could there be any potential conflict of interest?

In evaluating the worth of the research, remember you are being asked to review critically a study, or small group of studies. The exercise is therefore an analytical and evaluative one and not a descriptive one. The examiner will read the paper and will not expect the bulk of your critique to consist of a restatement of what the researchers did, how they did it and what their findings were. Although this can demonstrate some level of understanding of the study, you need to go well beyond this in evaluating the worth of the study.

Some initial questions about a study are these:

- Was the research placed within a sound theoretical background?
- Was an up-to-date and relevant review of previous work included in the introduction?
- Why was the study carried out?
- Was the research question sensibly and suitably framed?
- Were there clearly stated hypotheses being tested?

Your response to these questions will depend upon the context and nature of the research being considered. Thus the study may be novel and ground-breaking, but it should still have been conducted against a background of relevant previous work. Was an adequate justification for conducting the study made clear from the review of literature included in the paper? Not all studies have to state specific hypotheses being tested; although this is usually true of experimental studies, it may not be true of some exploratory descriptive ones such as surveys. Nevertheless, the aims and objectives of the research should always be clear.

Although the questions you will ask about a particular study and its methodology will depend upon the nature of the research, and will certainly be different for qualitative rather than quantitative papers, you may wish to approach a consideration of methodology with the following questions in mind:

- Was the study ethically acceptable and was ethical clearance obtained?
- Was the design of the study made clear in the description?
- Was the design of the study suitable for the question being investigated?
- How were participants selected and was the sampling method adequate?
- Was a pilot study conducted to establish a suitable number of participants and other aspects of methodology?

The design of a study should aim to minimise potential sources of bias, in the recruitment of subjects, in response rates to questionnaire or interview studies and in the way the study was conducted. If the researchers fail to provide important pieces of information – sometimes even the response rate in reports of surveys is omitted – you should be suspicious and not just assume that it is an oversight. The report of the methodology of a study should be in sufficient detail to enable another experienced researcher in the field to repeat the study in all its essential detail. This does not mean, given the practical consideration of the length of published papers, that every detail has to be specified; it is sufficient, for example, to refer to standard procedures which are used, as long as it is clear what was done.

Evaluating the adequacy of the data analysis is an area that requires careful thought and a good understanding of statistical or qualitative methods. In general, an assessment might bear the following questions in mind:

- Are the statistical or qualitative analyses that were conducted adequately described or referenced?
- Was the analysis appropriate for the design of the study?
- Is the presentation of the data in tables, charts, diagrams and so on clear and unambiguous?

Sometimes quite fundamental errors are made by researchers in analyses that have been carried out – such as statistical procedures inappropriate to the level of measurement of the variables employed. In the evaluation of a qualitative paper, was the process of data analysis a systematic one involving checks on the reliability and validity of the analysis, and what was the theoretical orientation for the analysis? Many procedures have passed under the rubric of qualitative analysis, where sometimes the researchers have done little more than establish a set of categories and counted up the number of responses falling into each.

An important part of any research paper is the discussion where the researchers draw conclusions from the findings. Here, you may wish to approach a critical reading of the discussion with the following questions uppermost in mind.

- Are the conclusions that are drawn from the findings fully justified?
- Are any limitations and weaknesses recognised by the researchers?
- Are the findings adequately discussed in the light of previous studies?

Overall, have the researchers tried to claim too much for the study in the light of what was done? A good discussion should adequately address the issue of generalisability of the findings in the context of the study design and difficulties encountered in practice. Finally, it should go without saying that the standard of referencing of the paper should be adequate; a list of references at the end should enable an interested reader to follow up other work in the field and check out methodological and other aspects of the study. Sometimes important references are omitted, or alternatively a paper may have too many references.

Chapter 18

I know there's an answer ...

The books in the lists which follow are concerned with various aspects of research methods and should prove helpful for students who are undertaking their research projects in the field of health. This is certainly not a comprehensive bibliography of the very many books on research methods of relevance to the field of health which have appeared over the years. Nor is it a 'personally recommended' selection; I have not read all the books listed here! However, whatever your specialised research project within the broad field of health, there should be some research methods volumes listed here which are of relevance and may be worth obtaining through the inter-library loans system if they are not available in your academic library.

Books on statistics are legion; unfortunately for the non-specialist, many can prove obscure or esoteric. For students completely new to the discipline of statistics, or who are unhappy with numerical concepts, I have found that the book by Francis Clegg provides a straightforward introduction to the basics; for a more advanced and comprehensive treatment of the subject from the health angle, the volume by Altman can be highly recommended. The classic text on non-parametric methods is provided by the Siegal and Castellan paperback although the more recent volume by Marjorie Pett is a more user-friendly text with examples specifically from the field of health. The SPSS software is commonly used in colleges and universities, the Bryman and Cramer book provides a readable guide to running most of the commonly used tests and the Kinnear and Gray is a widely used alternative.

Books on qualitative analysis can range from the basic to the highly technical; I have found that both Dey and Silverman provide readable no-nonsense introductions and the slim volume by Wolcot provides sound advice on reporting qualitative studies. The Miles and Huberman volume is a standard text on qualitative analysis which provides a very thorough review of the field. A very popular introductory guide to conducting a student research project is Judith Bell's book which uses examples from the educational field. The newer volume on research methods by Ann Bowling is recommended for its clarity and extensive use of examples from the field of health and health services research. The volume by Hart and Bond is an up-to-date introduction to the principles of 'real world' applied or action research in the health and social care fields.

Laboratory methods textbooks tend to be highly specialised, technical and expensive; I have listed some of relevance that I am aware of. The Sapsford and Abbott and the complementary reader by Abbott and Sapsford have proved popular with nursing students that I have taught as has the Parahoo volume, and the Coolican book is a very readable volume on psychological research methods. The McDowell and Newell volume is an excellent reference to many of the standard questionnaire instruments used by psychologists and health researchers. The later of the two volumes by Chalmers listed under Scientific Method and Philosophy is a thought provoking introduction to some theoretical positions on the nature of science and research enquiry and is valuable reading for any researcher.

Generic and miscellaneous research books

Anthony, D. (1996) *Health on the Internet*. Blackwell Science, Oxford.

Bailey, V. (1994) *Essential research skills*. Collins Educational.

Bell, J. (1999) *Doing your research project*. Open University Press, Buckingham.

Berg, K. and Latin, R.W. (1994) *Essentials of modern research methods in health, physical education and recreation*. Prentice Hall.

Bowling, A. (1997) *Measuring health: A review of quality of life measurement scales*. Open University Press, Buckingham.

Bowling, A. (1998) *Research methods in health: Investigating health and health services*. Open University Press, Buckingham.

Berge Britt-Marie, H.Ve. (2000) *Action research for gender equity*. Open University Press, Buckingham.

Brodie, B.A. (1998) *The ethics of biomedical research: An international perspective*. Oxford University Press.

Chalmers, I. and Altman, D. (1995) *Systematic reviews*. BMJ Books.

Cooksey, R.W. (1996) *Judgement analysis*. Academic Press, New York.

Crombie, I.K. (1996) *The pocket guide to critical appraisal*. BMJ Books.

Cryer, P. (1996) *The research student's guide to success*. Open University Press, Buckingham.

Day, A. (1998) *How to get research published in journals*. Gower Publishing.

De Konig, K. (1996) *Participatory research and health*. Zed Books.

Eichler, M. (1992) *Nonsexist research methods: A practical guide*. Routledge, London.

Fink, A. (1995) *How to design surveys*. Sage Publications, Thousand Oaks.

Graziano, A.M. (1997) *Research methods*. Scott, Foresman and Co.

Greenfield, T. (1996) *Research methods*. Edward Arnold Ltd.

Hall, G.M. (1998) *How to write a paper*. BMJ books.

Harding, S. (1987) *Feminism and methodology*. Indiana University Press.

Hart, C. (1998) *Doing a literature review*. Sage Publications, Thousand Oaks.

Kane, E. (1985) *Doing your own research*. Marion Boyers Publishers.

Kiley, R. (1996) *Medical information on the Internet*. Churchill Livingstone, Edinburgh.

Lee, R.M. (1993) *Doing research on sensitive topics*. Sage Publications, Thousand Oaks.

Lientz, B.P. and Rea, K.P. (1995) *Project management for the 21st century*. Academic Press, New York.

Litwin, M.S. (1995) *How to measure survey reliability and validity*. Sage Publications, Thousand Oaks.

Lock, S. and Wells, F. (1996) *Fraud and misconduct in medical research*. BMJ Books.

Lyver, D. and Swainson, G. (1995) *Basics of video production*. Butterworth-Heinemann,

Marshall, P. (1997) *Research methods: How to design and conduct a successful project*. How to Books Ltd.

Maynard, M. and Purvis, J. (1995) (Eds) *Researching women's lives from a feminist perspective*. Taylor and Francis, London.

McDowell, I. and Newell, C. (1996) *Measuring health: A guide to rating scales and questionnaires*. Oxford University Press.

McDowell, L., Race, P. and Brown, S. (1995) *500 tips for research students*. Kogan Page.

McNiff, J., Lomax, P. and Whitehead, J. (1996) *You and your action research project*. Routledge, Taylor and Francis.

Musgrave, J.R. (1996) *The digital scribe*. Academic Press, New York.

Peterson, R.A. (2000) *Constructing effective questionnaires*. Sage Publications, Thousand Oaks.

Petitti, D.B. (1994) *Meta-analysis, decision analysis and cost-effectiveness analysis*. Oxford University Press, Oxford.

Polgar, S. and Thomas, S.A. (1995) *Introduction to research in the health sciences.* Churchill Livingstone.

Ristock, J.L. and Pannell, J. (1997) *Community research as empowerment.* OUP, Canada.

Robson, C. (1993) *Real world research.* Blackwell, Oxford.

Sharp, J.A. and Howard, K. (1999) *The management of a student research project.* Gower Publishing, Aldershot.

Simmonds, D. and Reynolds, L. (1994) *Data presentation and visual literacy in medicine and science.* Butterworth-Heinemann.

Skeggs, B. (1997) *Formations of class and gender.* Sage Publications, London.

Smith, T. (1999) *Ethics in medical research: A handbook of good practice.* Cambridge University Press.

Stringer, E. T. (1999) *Action research.* Sage Publications, Thousand Oaks.

Tryfos, P. (1996) *Sampling methods for applied research.* John Wiley and Sons Ltd., Chichester.

Usherwood, T. (1999) *Introduction to project management in health research.* Open University Press, Buckingham.

Zeiger, M. (1999) *Essentials of writing biomedical research papers.* McGraw-Hill Health Professions Division.

Health services and health care research methods

Anderson, J.G. and Aydin, C.E. (1993) *Evaluating health care information systems.* Sage Publications, Newbury Park.

Black, N., Brazier, J., Reeve, B. and Fitzpatrick, R. (Eds) (1998) *Health services research methods.* Login Brothers Book Company.

Bowling, A. (1998) *Research methods in health.* Open University Press, Buckingham.

Colquhoun, D. and Kellehear, A. (1993) *Health research in practice: Political, ethical and methodological issues.* Chapman and Hall, London.

Daly, J., Willis, E. and McDonald, I. (1992) *Researching health care: Designs, dilemmas, disciplines.* Routledge, London.

Henry, I.C. (1995) *Community ethics and health care research.* Quay Books,

Heyman, B. (1995) *Researching user perspectives on community health care.* Chapman and Hall, London.

Lorig, K., Stewart, A., Ritter, P., Gonzaclez, V., Laurent, D. and Lynch, J. (1996) *Outcome measures for health education and other health care interventions.* Sage Publications, Newbury Park.

Loughlin, M. and Pashley, G. (1999) *Ethics of management in health care.* Butterworth-Heinemann,

Maynard, A. (1997) *Non-random reflections on health services research.* BMJ Publishing Group, London.

Munro, B.H. (1997) *Statistical methods for health care research.* Lippincott-Raven Publishers.

Ong, B.N. (1993) *Practice of health services research.* Chapman and Hall, London.

Open Learning Foundation (1996) *Inferential statistics in health care research.* Churchill Livingstone, New York.

Reid, N.G. (1992) *Health care research by degrees.* Blackwell Science Ltd., Oxford.

Ricketts, T.C. (1994) *Geographic methods for health services research: A focus on the rural-urban continuum.* University Press of America.

Sackett, D.L. (2000) *Evidence-based medicine.* Churchill Livingstone, Edinburgh.

St Leger, A.S. and Waisworth-Bell, J. (1999) *Change-promoting research for health services.* Open University Press, Buckingham.

Staquet, M.J., Hays, R.D. and Fayers, P.M. (Eds) (1998) *Quality of life assessment in clinical trials: Methods and practice.* Oxford University Press, Oxford.

Streiner, D.L. and Norman, G.R. (1996) *Health measurement scales: A practical guide to their development and use.* Oxford University Press, Oxford.

Laboratory and experimental research methods

Adolph, K.W. (Ed.) (1994) *Methods in molecular genetics*. Academic Press, New York.

Beesley, J.E. (1993) *Immunocytochemistry: A practical approach*. Oxford University Press, Oxford.

Bernard, C. (1999) *Experimental medicine*. Transaction Publishing.

Carpenter, R.H.S. and Robson, J.G. (Eds) (1999) *Vision research: A practical guide to laboratory methods*. Oxford University Press, Oxford.

Carson, P.A. and Dent, N.J. (1994) *Good laboratory and clinical practices*. Butterworth-Heinemann.

Castell, J.V. and Gomez-Lechon, M.J. (1996) *Methods in pharmaceutical research*. Academic Press, New York.

Cohen, J. and Wilkin, G.P. (Eds) (1996) *Neural cell culture: A practical approach*. Oxford University Press, Oxford.

Conn, P.M. and Sealfon, S.C. (1995) *Methods in neurosciences*. Academic Press, New York.

Davis, J.M. (Ed.) (1995) *Basic cell culture: A practical approach*. Oxford University Press, Oxford.

Fleiss, J.L. (1986) *The design and analysis of clinical experiments*. John Wiley and Sons Ltd, Chichester.

Fry, J.C. (Ed.) (1993) *Biological data analysis: A practical approach*. Oxford University Press, Oxford.

Glasel, J.A. and Deutscher, M.P. (1995) *Introduction to biophysical methods for protein and nucleic acid research*. Academic Press, New York.

Graham, J.M. and Rickwood, D. (1997) *Subcellular fractionation: A practical approach*. Oxford University Press, Oxford.

Haeckel, R. (Ed.) (1992) *Evaluation methods in laboratory medicine*. Wiley, Chichester.

Jennings, W., Mittlefehldt, E. and Stremple, P. (1997) *Analytical gas chromatography*. Academic Press, New York.

Kaufmann, S. and Kabelitz, D. (Eds) (1997) *Methods in microbiology*. Academic Press, New York.

Leftkovits, I. (1996) *Immunology methods manual*. Academic Press, New York.

Levy, E.R. and Herrington, C.S. (1995) *Non-isotopic methods in molecular biology: A practical approach*. Oxford University Press, Oxford.

Litten, R.Z. and Allen, J.P. (Eds) (1992) *Measuring alcohol consumption: Psychosocial and biochemical methods*. Humana Press.

Mahy, B.W.J. (Ed.) (1996) *Virology methods manual*. Academic Press, New York.

Malik, V.S. and Lillehoj, E.P. (1994) *Antibody techniques*. Academic Press, New York.

McKay, I. and Leigh, I. (1993) *Growth factors: A practical approach*. Oxford University Press, Oxford.

McNeill (Ed.) (1997) *Measurement of cardiovascular function*. CRC Press.

Monaco, A.P. (1995) *Pulsed field gel elecropheresis: A practical approach*. Oxford University Press, Oxford.

Ormerod, M.G. (1994) *Flow cytometry: A practical approach*. Oxford University Press, Oxford.

Reid, N. and Beesley, J.E. (1991) *Sectioning and cryosectioning for electron microscopy*. Elsevier, The Netherlands.

Reinhardt, C.A. (Ed.) (1994) *Alternatives to animal testing: New ways in the biomedical sciences, trends and progress*. Wiley, Chichester.

Seidman, L. and Moore, C. (1999) *Basic laboratory methods for biotechnology*. Prentice Hall, N.J.

Sugi, H. (Ed.) (1998) *Current methods in muscle physiology: Advantages, Problems and Limitations*. Oxford University Press, Oxford.

Thomas, J.A. (Ed.) (1996) *Endocrine methods*. Academic Press, New York.

Uhlig, S (Ed.) and Taylor, A.E. (1998) *Methods in pulmonary research*. Springer-Verlag.

Wolfc, R.R. (1992) *Radioactive and stable isotope tracers in biomedicine: Principles and practice of kinetic analysis*. Wiley, Chichester.

Wouterlood, F.G. (1995) *Neuroscience protocols, modules 1–4*. Elsevier, The Netherlands.

Yu, B.P. (Ed.) (1998) *Methods in aging research*. CRC Press.

Nursing and clinical research methods

Abbott, P. and Sapsford, R. (1997) *Research into practice: A reader for nurses and the caring professions.* Open University Press, Buckingham.

Armstrong, D. and Grace, J. (1995) *Research methods and audit in general practice.* Oxford University Press, Oxford.

Bailey, D.M. (1997) *Research for the health professional.* F.A. Davis and Co.

Brooker, C. and White, E. (1995) *Community psychiatric nursing: A research perspective.* Chapman and Hall, London.

Browner, W.S. and Hiscock, T. (1998) *Publishing and presenting clinical research.* Williams and Wilkins.

Burns, N. and Grove, S.K. (1996) *The practice of nursing research: Conduct, critique and utilization.* W.B. Saunders and Co.

Carter, Y. (1997) *Research methods in primary care.* Radcliffe Medical Press Ltd., Oxford.

Clifford, C. (1997) *Nursing and health care research: A skills-based introduction.* Prentice Hall.

Couchman, W. and Dawson, J. (1995) *Nursing and health-care research.* Scutari Press,

Crombie, L.E. with Davies, H.T.O. (1996) *Research in health care.* Wiley, Chichester.

Downey, P. (1997) *Homeopathy: A practical guide for the primary healthcare team.* Butterworth-Heinemann,

Drummond, A. (1996) *Research methods for therapists.* Chapman and Hall, London.

East, P. (1995) *Counselling in medical settings.* Open University Press, Buckingham.

Everitt, A., Hardiker, P., Littlewood, J. and Mullender, A. (1992) *Applied research for better practice.* Macmillan Press.

Fava, M. and Rosenbaum, J.F. (Eds) (1992) *Research designs and methods in psychiatry.* Elsevier, The Netherlands.

Field, P.A. and Morse, J.M. (1996) *Nursing research: The application of qualitative approaches.* Chapman and Hall, London.

Frank-Stromborg, M., Sharon, J. and Olsen, R. (1998) *Instruments for clinical health-care research.* Jones and Bartlett Publishing.

French, S. (1993) *Practical research: A guide for therapists.* Butterworth-Heinemann,

Gluekauf, R.L., Sechrest, L.B., Bond, G.R. and McDonel, E.C. (1993) *Improving assessment in rehabilitation and health.* Sage Publications, Newbury Park.

Hicks, C.M. (1995) *Research methods for physiotherapists.* Churchill Livingstone.

Higgs, J. and Jones, M. (1995) *Clinical reasoning in the health professions.* Butterworth-Heinemann,

Hoskins, C.N. (Ed.) (1998) *Developing research in nursing and health: Quantitative and qualitative methods.* Springer Publishing Company.

Jenkinson, C. (1997) *Assessment and evaluation of heath and medical care.* Open University Press, Buckingham.

Lobiondo-Wood, G. and Haber, J. (1997) *Nursing research.* Mosby, London.

McLeod, J. (1994) *Doing counselling research.* Sage Publications, Thousand Oaks.

Morse, J.M. and Field, P.A. (1996) *Nursing research: The application of qualitative approaches.* Chapman and Hall, London.

Muller, D.J., Harris, P.J., Wattley, L. and Taylor, J. (1992) *Nursing children: Psychology, research and practice.* Chapman and Hall, London.

Ogles, B. M., Lambert, M.J. and Masters, K.S. (1996) *Assessing outcome in clinical practice.* Allyn and Bacon.

Open Learning Foundation (1996) *Qualitative research methodology in nursing and health care.* Churchill Livingstone, New York.

Parahoo, K. (1997) *Nursing research: Principles, process and issues.* Macmillan Press. London.

Reed, J. and Proctor, S. (1995) *Practitioner research in health care: The inside story.* Chapman and Hall, London.

Polit-O'Hara, D., Hungler, B. and Polit, D. (1998) *Nursing research: Principles and methods.* Lippincott Williams & Wilkins Publishers.

Sapsford, R. and Abbott, P. (1992) *Research methods for nurses and the caring professions.* Open University Press, Buckingham.

Simon, A. and Boyer, E. (1975) *The reflective practitioner.* Basic Books, New York.

Smith, P. (1997) *Research mindedness for practice.* Churchill Livingstone, London.

Smith, P. (1998) *Nursing research.* Arnold.

Psychological research methods

Aiken, L.R. (1996) *Questionnaires and inventories: Surveying opinions and assessing personality.* Wiley, Chichester.

Aiken, L.R. (1996) *Rating scales and checklists: Evaluating behaviour, personality and attitudes.* Wiley, Chichester.

Algom, D. (Ed.) (1992) *Psychophysical approaches to cognition.* Elsevier, The Netherlands.

Allen, J.D. and Pittenger, D.J. (1991) *Statistics tutor: Tutorial and computational software for the behavioural sciences,* student edition. Wiley, Chichester.

Barker, C. (1994) *Research methods in clinical and counselling psychology.* Wiley, Chichester.

Breakwell, G. (1995) *Research methods in psychology.* Sage Publications, Newbury Park.

Cacioppo, J.T., Judd, C.M. and Reis, H.T. (Eds) (2000) *Handbook of research methods in social and personality psychology.* Cambridge University Press.

Caverni, J.P., Fabre, J.M. and Gonzalez, M. (Eds) (1990) *Cognitive biases.* Elsevier, The Netherlands.

Colman, A. (Ed.) (1995) *Psychological research methods and statistics.* Addison-Wesley Longman Ltd.

Coolican, H. (1996) *Introduction to research methods and statistics in psychology.* Hodder and Stoughton, London.

Cozby, P.C. (1996) *Methods in behavioural research.* Mayfield Publishing Company.

Edelmann, R.J. (1995) *Anxiety: Theory, research and intervention in clinical and health psychology.* John Wiley and Sons Ltd., Chichester.

Elson-Cook, T.M. and Moyse, R. (1992) *Knowledge negotiation.* Academic Press, New York.

Eye, A.E. (1996) *Categorical variables in developmental research.* Academic Press, New York.

Goodwin, C.J. (1998) *Research in psychology: Methods and design.* Wiley, Chichester.

Grimm, L.G. (1993) *Statistical applications for the behavioural sciences.* Wiley, Chichester.

Heiman. G.W. (1998) *Research methods in psychology.* Houghton Mifflin.

Iversen, I.H. and Lattal, K.A. (Eds) (1991) *Experimental analysis of behaviour.* Elsevier, The Netherlands.

Maxwell, D.L. (1997) *Research and statistical methods in communication disorders.* Williams and Wilkins Co.

Minium, E.W. and King, B.M. (1993) *Statistical reasoning in psychology and education.* Wiley, Chichester.

Reaves, C.C. (1991) *Quantitative research for the behavioural sciences.* Wiley, Chichester.

Richardson, J. (1996) *Handbook of qualitative research methods for psychology and the social sciences.* DCLP Publishers.

Schaughnessy, J.J., Zechmeister, E.B. and Zechmeister, J.S. (1996) *Research methods in psychology.* McGraw-Hill Book Co.

Schweigert, W.A. (1994) *Research methods and statistics for psychology.* Wadsworth Publishing Co.

Sheldon, B. (1995) *Cognitive-behavioural therapy: Research, practice and philosophy.* Routledge, London.

Stemmer, B. (1997) *Handbook of neurolinguistics.* Academic Press, New York.

Stone, H. and Sidel, J. (1992) *Sensory evaluation practices.* Academic Press, New York.

Summers, J.J. (Ed.) (1992) *Approaches to the study of motor control and learning.* Elsevier, The Netherlands.

Thomas, J.R. and Nelson, J.K. (1996) *Research methods in physical activity.* Human Kinetics.

Whittle, M.W. (1996) *Gait analysis.* Heinemann.

Vadum, A. C. and Rankin, N.O. (1997) *Psychological research: Methods for discovery and validation.* McGraw-Hill College Division.

Van Someren, M.W., Barnard and Y.F., Sandberg, J.A.C. (1994) *The think aloud method: A practical guide to modelling cognitive processes.* Academic Press, New York.

Zechmeister, E.B. (1996) *Practical introduction to research methods in psychology.* McGraw-Hill Book Co.

Qualitative research methods

Agar, M.H. (1996) *The professional stranger: An informal introduction to ethnography.* Academic Press, New York.

Atkinson, P. and Hammersley, M. (1995) *Ethnography: Principles in practice.* Routledge, London.

Barbour, R. S. and Kitzinger, J. (1998) *Developing focus group research.* Sage Publications, Thousand Oaks.

Berg, B.L. (1997) *Qualitative research methods for the social sciences.* Allyn and Bacon Ltd.

Bornal, J. (1999) *Biographical interviews: Link between research and practice.* Centre for Policy on Ageing.

Brenner, M., Brown, J. and Canter, D. (1985) *The research interview: Uses and approaches.* Academic Press, New York.

Coffey, A. (1999) *The ethnographic self.* Sage Publications, Thousand Oaks.

Crabtree, B.F. and Miller, W.L. (1999) *Doing qualitative research.* Sage Publications, Thousand Oaks.

Denzin, N.K. and Lincoln, Y.S. (1998) *Collecting and interpreting qualitative materials.* Sage Publications, Thousand Oaks.

Dey, I. (1993) *Qualitative data analysis.* Routledge, London.

Fielding, N.G. and Lee, R. M. (1996) *Computer analysis and qualitative research.* Sage Publications, Thousand Oaks.

Gilgun, J.F. (1992) *Qualitative methods in family research.* Sage Publications, Newbury Park.

Greenbaum, T.L. (1988) *The practical handbook and guide to focus group research.* Lexington Press, Lexington, MA.

Gubrium, J.F. (1994) *Qualitative methods in aging research.* Sage Publications, Newbury Park.

Gubrium, J.F. and Holstein, J.A. (1997) *The new language of qualitative method.* Oxford University Press, Oxford.

Hammersley, M. (1992) *What's wrong with ethnography?* Routledge, London.

Krueger, R.A. (1994) *Focus groups: A practical guide for applied research.* Sage Publications, Thousand Oaks.

Kvale, S. (1996) *Interviews: An introduction to qualitative research interviewing.* Sage Publications, Thousand Oaks.

Lawler, R.W. and Carley, K.M. (1996) *Case study and computing: Advanced qualitative methods in the study of human behaviour.* Intellect Publications, USA.

Mays, N. (1996) *Qualitative research in health care.* BMJ Publishing Group, London.

Merton, R.K., Fiske, M. and Kendall, P.L. (1990) *The focussed interview.* Free Press, New York.

Miles, M.B. and Huberman A.M. (1994) *Qualitative data analysis.* Sage Publications, Thousand Oaks.

Morgan, D.L. (1993) *Successful focus groups.* Sage Publications, Newbury Park.

Morse, J.M. (1992) *Qualitative health research.* Sage Publications, Newbury Park.

Naumes, W. and Naumes, M.J. (1999) *The art and craft of case writing.* Sage Publications, Thousand Oaks.

Patton, M.Q. (1990) *Qualitative evaluation and research methods.* Sage Publications, Newbury Park.

Ribbens, J. and Edwards, R. (1997) *Feminist dilemmas in qualitative research*. Sage Publications, Thousand Oaks.

Rubin, H.J. and Rubin, I.S. (1995) *Qualitative interviewing*. Sage Publications, Newbury Park.

Silverman, D. (1993) *Interpreting qualitative data*. Sage Publications, London.

Silverman, D. (1999) *Doing qualitative research: A practical handbook*. Sage Publications, Thousand Oaks.

Spradley, J.P. (1979) *The ethnographic interview*. Holt, Reinhardt and Winston, New York.

Stake, R. E. (1995) *The art of case study research*. Sage Publications, Thousand Oaks.

Strauss, A. and Corbin, J. (1997) *Grounded theory in practice*. Sage Publications, Thousand Oaks.

Strauss, A. and Corbin, J. (1999) *Basics of qualitative research*. Sage Publications, Thousand Oaks.

Walker, R. and Schratz, M. (1995) *Research as social change: New opportunities for qualitative research*. Routledge, London.

Weber, R.P. (1985) *Basic content analysis*. Sage Publications, Beverly Hills, CA.

Wolcot, H.F. (1990) *Writing up qualitative research*. Sage University Paper, Newbury Park.

Yin, R.K. (1993) *Applications of case study research*. Sage Publications, Thousand Oaks.

Scientific method and philosophy

Agnew, N.M and Pyke, S.W. (1991) *The science game*. Prentice-Hall, Englewood Cliffs, NJ.

Appleyard, B. (1992) *Understanding the present: Science and the soul of modern man*. Picador.

Atkinson, T. and Claxton, G. (Eds) (2000) *The intuitive practitioner: On the value of not always knowing what one is doing*. Open University Press, Buckingham.

Barnes, B., Bloor, D. and Henry, J. (Eds) (1996) *Scientific knowledge: A sociological analysis*. University of Chicago Press.

Carey, J. (1996) *The Faber book of science*. Faber.

Chalmers, A.F. (1990) *Science and its fabrication*. Open University Press, Buckingham.

Chalmers, A.F. (1992) *What is this thing called science?* Open University Press, Buckingham.

Fenstad, J.E., Frolov, I.T. and Hilpinen, R. (Eds) (1989) *Logic, methodology and philosophy of science VIII*. Elsevier, The Netherlands.

Illich, I. (1991) *Limits to medicine*. Penguin Books, Harmondsworth.

Latour, B. and Woolgar, S. (1986) *Laboratory life: The construction of scientific facts*. Princeton University Press.

Longino, H.E. (1990) *Science as social knowledge: Values and objectivity in scientific inquiry*. Princeton University Press.

Reason, P. and Rowan, J.L. (1987) *Human enquiry: A source book of new paradigm research*. Wiley, London.

Wolpert, L. (1992) *The unnatural nature of science*. Faber Books.

Social research methods

Adey, L. A. (1996) *Designing and conducting health surveys: A comprehensive guide*. Jossey-Bass Publishers.

Baldwin, S. (1997) *Needs assessment and community care*. Butterworth-Heinemann.

Bickman, L. and Rog, D.J. (1997) *Handbook of applied social research methods*. Sage Publications, Newbury Park.

Bulmer, M. (Ed.) (1999) *Sociological research methods*. Macmillan Ltd. and Transaction Publishers.

Chen, S. (1998) *Mastering research: A guide to the methods of social and behavioural sciences*. Burnham Inc. Publishing.

Chignell, H. (1990) *Data in sociology*. Causeway Press.

De Vijer, F.J.R. (1997) *Methods and data analysis for cross-cultural research*. Alta Mira Press.

Fink, A., Fielder, E. P. and Frey, J.H. (1995) *The survey handbook*. Sage Publications, Newbury Park.

Frankfort-Nachmias, C. (1996) *Research methods in the social sciences*. Edward Arnold Ltd.

Greenacre, M. (1994) *Correspondence analysis in the social sciences*. Academic Press, New York.

Greif, G.L. and Ephross, P.H. (1997) *Group work with populations at risk*. Oxford University Press, Oxford.

Hantrais, L. (1996) *Cross-national research methods in the social sciences*. Pinter Publishers Ltd.

Hart, E. and Bond, M. (1995) *Action research for health and social care: A guide to practice*. Open University Press, Buckingham.

Hayashi, C., Suzuki, T. and Sasaki, M. (1992) *Data analysis for comparative social research*. Elsevier, The Netherlands.

Hinton, P.R. (1995) *Statistics explained: A guide for social science students*. Routledge, London.

Huber, G. (1995) *Longitudinal field research methods*. Sage Publications, Newbury Park.

McNeill, P. (1990) *Research methods*. Routledge and Kegan Paul, London.

Moustakas, C. (1994) *Phenomenological research methods*. Sage Publications, Newbury Park.

Namboodiri, K. (1994) *Methods for macrosociological research*. Academic Press, New York.

Neuman, W.L. (1994) S*ocial research methods: Qualitative and quantitative approaches*. Allyn and Bacon Inc.

Reinharz, S. (1992) *Feminist methods in social research*. Oxford University Press, Oxford.

Ristock, J.L. and Pennell, J. (1997) *Community research as empowerment*. Oxford University Press, Oxford.

Robinson, D. and Reed, V. (1997) *A-Z of social research jargon*. Arena.

Singleton, R.A., Straits, B.C. and Straits, M.M. (1993) *Approaches to social research*. Oxford University Press, Oxford.

Sanger, J. (1996) *The complete observer: A field research guide to observation*. Falmer Press, London.

Stanfield, J.H. and Dennis, R.M. (Ed.) (1993) *Race and ethnicity in research methods*. Sage Publications, Newbury Park.

Statistics and epidemiological research methods

Abrahamson, J.H. (1994) *Making sense of data*. Oxford University Press, Oxford.

Altman, D.G. (1991) *Practical statistics for medical research*. Chapman and Hall.

Armitage, P. (1994) *Statistical methods in medical research*. Blackwell Science Ltd., Oxford.

Blasius, J. (1997) *Visualization of categorical data*. Academic Press, New York.

Brown, R.A. and Swanson Beck, J. (1994) *Medical statistics on personal computers: A guide to the appropriate use of statistics packages*. BMJ Publishing Group, London.

Bryman, A. and Cramer, D. (1999) *Quantitative data analysis with SPSS for Windows*. Routledge, London.

Bruce, N. (1995) *Research and change in urban community health*. Avebury Publishing Co. Ltd.

Campbell, M.J. and Machin, D. (1993) *Medical statistics: A commonsense approach*. Wiley, Chichester.

Clegg, F. (1992) *Simple statistics*. Cambridge University Press.

Cramer, D. (1997) *Basic statistics for social research*. Routledge, London.

Dean, K. (1993) *Population health research*. Sage Publications, Newbury Park.

Dixon, R.A., Munro, J.F. and Silcocks, P.B. (1997) *The evidence based medicine workbook*. Butterworth Heinemann.

Everitt, B.S. (1992) *The analysis of contingency tables*. Chapman and Hall, London.

Fink, A. (1995) *How to analyze survey data*. Sage Publications, Thousand Oaks.

Foster, J. (1996) *Data analysis using SPSS for Windows*. Sage Publications, Thousand Oaks.

Frank, I.E. and Todeschini, R. (1994) *The data analysis handbook*. Elsevier, The Netherlands.

Freund, R.J. and Wilson, W.J. (1998) *Regression analysis*. Academic Press, New York.

Ghosh, S. and Rao, C.R. (Eds) (1996) *Handbook of statistics 13: Design and analysis of experiments*. Elsevier, The Netherlands.

Jadad, A. R. (1998) *Randomised controlled trials*. BMJ Books.

Kahn, H.A. and Sempos, C.T. (1989) *Statistical methods in epidemiology*. Oxford University Press, Oxford.

Kelsey, J.L., Whittemore, A.S., Evans, A.S. and Thompson, W.D. (1996) *Methods in observational epidemiology*. Oxford University Press, Oxford.

Kinnear, P.R. and Gray, C.D. (1994) *SPSS for Windows made simple*. Lawrence Erlbaum Associates, Hove.

Kline, P. (1994) *An easy guide to factor analysis*. Routledge, London.

Kleinbaum, D.G. (1994) *Logistic regression: A self-learning text.* Springer-Verlag.

Kleinbaum, D.G. (Ed.) (1997) *Applied regression analysis and other multivariable methods.* Duxbury Publishing.

Korn, E. L. and Graubard, B.I. (1999) *Analysis of health surveys.* John Wiley and Sons Ltd., Chichester.

Mark, J. (1998) *Critical appraisal of epidemiological studies and clinical trials*. Oxford University Press, Oxford.

McNeil, D. (1996) *Epidemiological research methods.* John Wiley and Sons Ltd., Chichester.

Norusis, M.J. (1994) *SPSS for Windows base system user's guide*. SPSS Inc.

Norusis, M.J. (1994) *SPSS Advanced Statistics*. SPSS Inc.

Pett, M.A. (1997) *Nonparametric statistics for health care research*. Sage Publications, Thousand Oaks.

Rao, C.R. (Ed.) (1993) *Multivariate analysis; Future directions*. Elsevier, The Netherlands.

Rao, C.R. and Chakraborty, R. (Eds) (1991) *Handbook of statistics 8: Statistical methods in biological and medical sciences.* Elsevier, The Netherlands.

Rovine, M.J. and Von Eye, A. (1991) *Applied computational statistics in longitudinal research.* Academic Press, New York.

Siegal, S. and Castellan, N. J. (1988) *Nonparametric statistics*. McGraw Hill International.

Staquet, M., Hays, R. and Fayers, P. (Eds) (1998) *Quality of life assessment in clinical trials.* Oxford University Press, Oxford.

Unwin, N., Carr, S. and Leeson, J. (1997) *An introductory study guide to public health and epidemiology*. Open University Press, Buckingham.

Von Eye, A. (Ed.) (1990) *New statistical methods in longitudinal research*. Academic Press, New York.

Wilcox, R.R. (1995) *Statistics for the social sciences*. Academic Press, New York.

And finally...

Do not be apprehensive because you may be conducting a substantial piece of research for the first time; doing good research is *never* easy and it is recognised that student projects are likely to contain flaws. Many experienced researchers find that they make errors in the way they go about their activities. Research is an exciting, creative and rewarding process, although it needs to be said that it can also be very frustrating and normally involves much routine legwork. In fact, students who register for research (higher) degrees are being assessed as much on their perseverance and 'stickability' as on their academic ability. Remember also that the research is essentially under your own control but that things are likely to, and often do, go wrong. People do not turn up for interviews, refusals are encountered and sometimes ethics committees turn down carefully worked out proposals for apparently bureaucratic reasons.

In order to circumvent such obstacles, you will need to commit time and application to planning for all contingencies; carefully planning a project is at least half the battle. As I have been concerned to emphasise, much of the rest can be tackled by a methodical and disciplined attitude to the work you conduct. You will probably also need to be prepared to compromise, for research is often a pragmatic activity. However, do not always be tempted to take the easy route in your research. You should know enough by now to recognise the limitations of convenience samples by comparison with true random samples, and be prepared to discuss if necessary the representative nature of people who have been stopped in the street compared to the population of interest in your discussion of your findings.

Above all, if I can give you one piece of advice which should be borne in mind in planning your project, it is this. Do not be tempted to be over-ambitious in what you attempt to achieve. It is a temptation to pose an interesting and important question in your research but not to be able to answer it properly, given the strictly limited time and resources at your disposal in an undergraduate project. It is far better to formulate a straightforward, simple question which can be answered within these limitations than to attempt something more profound and wide ranging which, in research terms, will be inadequately addressed. I cannot put it better than one author, David Silverman, who has written as follows:

> it is important to find the causes of a social problem like homelessness, but such a problem is beyond the scope of a single researcher with limited time and resources. Moreover, by defining the problem so widely, one is usually unable to say anything in great depth about it. As I tell my students, your aim should be to say 'a lot about a little (problem)'. This means avoiding the temptation to say 'a little about a lot'. Indeed the

latter path can be something of a 'cop-out'. Precisely because the topic is so wide-ranging, one can flit from one aspect to another without being forced to refine and test each piece of analysis.'

(Silverman 1993:3)

Good luck with your project!

Choosing and using a computer for research

There is little doubt that the personal computer has proved the most valuable general purpose research tool which has appeared in recent decades. Prior to the personal computer revolution, which gathered pace in the 1980s and flourished in the 1990s, researchers were tied to generally unfriendly multi-user mainframe based systems accessed via terminals in universities and host institutions. In the twenty-first century, the personal computer gives the lone researcher working at home, or in the field with a laptop PC, the facilities and power, through user-friendly menu driven software, of data processing and analysis which was only dreamt of for most of the twentieth century.

Microcomputer power doubles about every eighteen months, so I am conscious that any advice given about microcomputer hardware, or indeed software, becomes out of date almost as soon as it is written. However, some general principles have stood the test of time. It is generally true that the faster and more sophisticated the computer you buy, the longer will be its useful effective life before the increasing demands of software development render it inadequate. Having said this, and given the limited funds of many students, it is not necessary to buy the latest and fastest multi-media wonder for the purposes of assisting a research study. Thus, at the time of writing, computers running at over 900MHz with 512Mb RAM (memory) and 30Gb (gigabyte) or more of hard disk storage are at the leading edge of home computer technology. A machine of less than half this processor speed with 64Mb RAM (or 128Mb for Windows 2000) is perfectly adequate for most applications. Commonly used research software is generally not graphics intensive, as games are, and there is little or no need to purchase a machine with this capability. At the time of writing, a used Pentium PC which will adequately run all the required software can be purchased for a couple of hundred pounds or so. A 2Gb or larger hard disk capacity is sufficient to install all the software listed below and still provide adequate room for data files. A PC with a CD-ROM drive is almost an essential requirement now since most software is distributed using this medium, but the more expensive DVD drive is not necessary on a research machine.

The software you may consider it helpful to acquire, and which will handle over 95 per cent of most research project needs, includes:

- Microsoft Windows 95 or higher operating system
- a web browser
- a word processing package
- a spreadsheet
- a presentation graphics package
- a statistical analysis package
- a qualitative analysis package.

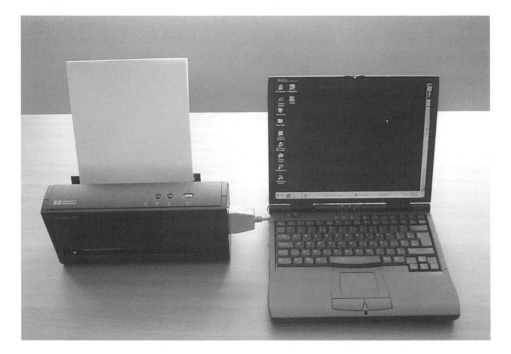

Figure A1.1 A modern laptop PC with a portable ink-jet printer.

Other software that can be helpful for research purposes includes database management software, desktop publishing software, project management software and specialist 'vertical market' applications such as packages to assist with the calculation of sample sizes and confidence limits.

As software has become more standardised in recent years with the almost universal adoption of the Microsoft Windows operating systems on personal computers, software compatibility has become less of an issue than once it was. Thus most word processing packages will enable you to save a file as an RTF (rich text format) file which can be read by almost any version of a variety of word processing packages, retaining the bulk of the special formatting features in the original file. Later versions of software packages tend to be 'backwards compatible' with earlier versions, although earlier versions may not be able to read the file structure of the latest version. The moral here is that it is not always necessary to use the latest versions of software so long as the file is saved either in a 'portable' format such as RTF or in a version that can be read by any generation of the software. Data entry, for example, can be achieved quite easily and efficiently using the Excel 3 spreadsheet file format and this can be read by any later version of Excel as well as other packages, such as most versions of the SPSS (Statistical Package for the Social Sciences) software. Earlier versions of industry standard, or compatible, software can often be obtained very cheaply from discount sources, or may be given away as cover disks on computer magazines. It is also worth mentioning that companies like Microsoft and SPSS Inc. sometimes offer substantial special educational discounts for their software to students.

Access to the internet is provided by a modem and a suitable web browser as discussed in

Chapter 12. Although at the time of writing a 56K dial-up modem is the standard means of internet access, this is likely to change radically with the emergence of broadband technologies. The 56K maximum speed is limited by the copper telephone lines connecting homes to telephone exchanges, although digital broadband access through telephone sockets is likely to revolutionise internet connection speeds in the next few years. This is an important practical point, since accessing graphics intensive sites and downloading files can be a lengthy and unreliable process with 56K modem technology.

It is good practice to try a computer before you buy; keyboards may be less variable in quality than they used to be but there are still significant differences in the 'feel' of keyboards. The quality of the monitor in particular is an important factor that can only be determined by inspection. A 'fuzzy' monitor or one that flickers, even almost imperceptibly, can cause eye-strain and be tiring to use for extended periods. Non-interlaced screens with a minimum refresh rate of 72Hz are recommended.

A printer is an almost essential adjunct to a PC. The choice of printer is governed by a number of factors, including speed, quality, running costs and ease of obtaining consumables. Although colour ink-jet printers are a popular choice, the cost per page is much higher than a basic monochrome laser printer for around the same price. The latter is suitable for almost any task except the production of colour overhead transparencies for presentations and colour charts in reports. Other types of printer, including dot matrix types, are now outdated and should be avoided. Cheap special offer printers may turn out to be less than good value if the consumables (such as cartridges) are expensive or hard to obtain.

Laptop computers have the advantage of being usable in the field almost anywhere on battery power, and this can be an important factor for some projects. Data entry can be achieved at the same time as collection using a laptop and suitable software. A laptop and a portable battery-operated printer, as is shown in Figure A1.1, can provide complete office facilities in the field. However, laptops are more expensive than their desktop equivalents, can be expensive to repair should they go wrong and can be difficult or impossible to upgrade like desktop PCs which generally use standard parts. Should funds be limited, go for a desktop model instead and be prepared to forgo the convenience and cachet of carrying around a laptop.

Internet addresses to get started

- All the internet addresses below have the initial prefix http://
- World wide web addresses start with the subsequent prefix www
- Gopher addresses start with a different subsequent prefix indicated below.
- All the addresses below were active and functional at the time of writing, but some addresses may change over time.

Academic Press journals online	gort.ucsd.edu/newjour/search.html
American Cancer Society	www.cancer.org/frames.html
American Medical Association	www.ama-assn.org/
American Nurses Association	www.ana.org/
American Sociological Review	www.pop.psu.edu/ASR/asr.htm
Annual Reviews of Biomedical Sciences	biomedical.annualreviews.org/
Audit Commission	www.audit-commission.gov.uk/
BIDS	www.bids.ac.uk/
Biotechnology and Biological Sciences Research Council	www.bbsrc.ac.uk/
Blackwell's Bookshop	www.blackwell.co.uk/bookshops/
British Association of Occupational Therapists	www.cot.co.uk/
British Broadcasting Corporation	www.bbc.co.uk/
British Journal of Clinical Psychology	journals.eecs.qub.ac.uk/BPS/BJCP/BJCP.html
British Journal of Health Psychology	journals.eecs.qub.ac.uk/BPS/BJHP/BJHP.html
British Journal of Medical Psychology	journals.eecs.qub.ac.uk/BPS/BJMP/BJMP.html
British Journal of Psychology	journals.eecs.qub.ac.uk/BPS/BJP/BJP.html
British Journal of Social Psychology	journals.eecs.qub.ac.uk/BPS/BJSP/BJSP.html
British Journal of Sociology	www.lse.ac.uk/serials/bjs/
British Library	portico.bl.uk/
British Medical Association	www.bma.org.uk/
British Medical Journal	www.bmj.com/index.shtml
British Psychological Society	www.bps.org.uk/
Brunel Health Economics Research Group	http1.brunel.ac.uk:8000/depts/herg/
Butterworth-Heinemann publishers	www.butterworth.heinemann.co.uk/
Cambridge University Press	www.cup.cam.ac.uk/
Cardiff University	www.cf.ac.uk/
Centre for advanced research in phenomenology	www.flinet.com/~corp/
Centre for Disease Control	hwcweb.hwc.ca/hpb/lcdc/hp_eng.html

Cochrane abstracts of reviews	www.update-software.com/abstracts/
Communicable Disease Surveillance Centre	www.open.gov.uk/doh/dhhome.htm
Cornell University	www.cornell.edu/
CTI centre for sociology, politics and social policy	www.stir.ac.uk/socinfo/
Department of Health	www.open.gov.uk/doh/dhhome.htm
DoctorsNet UK	www.doctors.net.uk/
Engineering and Science Research Council	www.esrc.ac.uk/
English National Board for Nursing, Midwifery and Health Visiting	www.enb.org.uk/
European centre for social research and policy	www.euro.centre.org/causa/ec/
European Research Group on Health Outcomes	www.meb.uni-bonn.de/standards/ERGHO/
Evidence-based health links	nzhta.chmeds.ac.nz/links/evidence.htm
Federation of American Societies for Experimental Biology	www.faseb.org/
Galaxy Medicine	galaxy.einet.net/galaxy/Medicine.html
Grounded theory methodology on the web	gtm.nawala.net/gtm-19.html
Grounded Theory Institute	www.groundedtheory.com/
Guardian, The	www.guardian.co.uk/
Hansard	www.parliament.thestationery-office.co.uk/pa/cm/cmhansrd.htm
Harvard University	www.harvard.edu/
Health Economics Research Unit	www.abdn.ac.uk/public_health/heru/index.html
Health Education Authority	www.hea.org.uk/index.html
Health Education Board for Scotland	www.hebs.org.uk/
Health Promotion Information Centre	www.hea.org.uk/hpic
Health Promotion Wales	www.hpw.org.uk/
Health Service Management Centre	www.bham.ac.uk/hsmc/
Health Service Journal	www.hsj.co.uk/
Health Services Research Journal	www.xnet.com/~hnet/hsr.htm
Health Matters	www.bbc.co.uk/worldservice/healthmatters/
Healthworks online	www.healthworks.co.uk/
Independent, The	www.Independent.co.uk/
Imperial Cancer Research Fund	www.icnet.uk/
Infoseek health channel	www.infoseek.co.uk/Health
Institute of Health Sciences	www.his.ox.ac.uk/
John Wiley publishers	www.wiley.co.uk
Journal of the American Medical Association	www.ama-assn.org/public/journals/jama/
Journal of Biochemistry	www.portlandpress.co.uk/bj/
Journal of Physiology	physiology.cup.cam.ac.uk/Jphysiol/
Kings Fund	www.kingsfund.org.uk/
Library of Congress	lcweb.loc.gov/
Lippincott's Nursing Center	www.nursingcenter.com/
Medical Research Council	www.nimr.mrc.ac.uk/MRC/home.html
Medline	www4.ncbi.nlm.nih.gov/PubMed/
Medscape (UK)	www.medscape.com
MedWeb	medweb.bham.ac.uk/
MIDAS population statistics	midas.ac.uk
Ministry of Agriculture, Fisheries and Food	www.maff.gov.uk
National Electronic Library for Health	www.nelh.nhs.uk/
National Electronic Library for Mental Health	cebmh.warne.ox.ac.uk/cebmh/nelmh/

National Library of Medicine	www.nlm.nih.gov/
National Research Register	www.update-software.com/nrronline/NRROpen.htm
Nature	www.nature.com/
New Scientist	www.newscientist.com/
NHS Confederation	www.nhsconfed.net/
NHS Information Authority	www.nhsia.nhs.uk/
NISS (Networked Information Systems)	niss.ac.uk/
Nuffield Institute for Health	www.leeds.ac.uk/nuffield/home.html
Nursing journals online	medweb.bham.ac.uk/nursing/journals
Nursing Standard online	www.nursing-standard.co.uk
Nursing Times	med714.bham.ac.uk/nursing/journals/nursing-times.html
OMNI health information	www.omni.ac.uk/
Open University	www.open.ac.uk
Open University Press	www.openup.ac.uk/
Oxford Centre for Evidence-based Medicine	cebm.jr2.ox.ac.uk/
Oxford University	ww.ox.ac.uk/
Oxford University Press	www.oup.co.uk/
Patient UK	www.patient.co.uk/
Penguin books	www.penguin.com
Physiotherapy Evidence Database (PEDRO)	ptwww.cchs.usyd.edu.au/pedro/
PORTICO (British Library)	portico.bl.uk/
Public Health Laboratory Service	www.phls.co.uk/
RAND Corporation	www.rand.org/
Routledge publishers	www.routledge.com
Royal Statistical Society	www.maths.ntu.ac.uk/rss/index.html
Sage publications	www.sageltd.co.uk/
Scientific American	www.sciam.com
Silverplatter	www.silverplatter.com/
Social Science and Medicine	www.elsevier.nl:80/inca/publications/store/3/1/5/
Social Science Information Gateway	sosig.ac.uk/
Sociology gopher resources	gopher://marvel.loc.gov:70/11/global/socsci/soc
Sociosite	www.pscw.uva.nl/sociosite/TOPICS/index.html
SPSS Inc.	www.spss.com/
Statistics on the web	www.execpc.com/~helberg/statistics.html
The Lancet	www.thelancet.com
Times, The	www.the_times.co.uk/
Turning Research into Practice Database	www.ceres.uwcm.ac.uk/
UK central government information	bubl.ac.uk/uk/government.htm
UK practice guidelines database	www.ihs.ox.ac.uk/guidelines/index.html
University of Bristol	www.bris.ac.uk/
University of Cambridge	www.cam.ac.uk/
University of Edinburgh	www.ed.ac.uk/
University of Essex data archives	www.essex.ac.uk/
University of Glasgow	www.gla.ac.uk/
University of Leeds	www.leeds.ac.uk/
University of Liverpool	www.liv.ac.uk/
University of London	www.lon.ac.uk
University of York, Centre for Reviews and Dissemination	www.york.ac.uk/np.deptindex.htm#research
Wellcome Trust	www.wellcome.ac.uk/w2rr.html
World Health Organisation	www.who.ch/

Random numbers

Table AIII.1 can be helpful whenever subjects need to be drawn randomly from lists, for the allocation of groups in experimental work, or whenever a process of randomisation is called for. The use of this table is explained in Chapter 4.

Table AIII.1 1000 random numbers from 0 to 1

0.7229	0.9049	0.8477	0.0350	0.4904	0.2329	0.3750	0.9980
0.9325	0.1853	0.4403	0.9640	0.7214	0.3360	0.0973	0.0749
0.4240	0.1078	0.1676	0.5369	0.4271	0.3574	0.9036	0.1181
0.9876	0.2899	0.5534	0.0809	0.3407	0.2971	0.2950	0.2242
0.5074	0.0133	0.5776	0.5416	0.4471	0.9656	0.8480	0.6406
0.3996	0.3689	0.5723	0.7257	0.7558	0.8571	0.2524	0.2617
0.5066	0.9383	0.9187	0.8413	0.2464	0.1081	0.8955	0.7577
0.9810	0.4624	0.4303	0.5922	0.6132	0.0037	0.3227	0.1937
0.8147	0.3536	0.5124	0.9523	0.8877	0.8589	0.6137	0.3662
0.9012	0.4193	0.2879	0.8230	0.4228	0.6452	0.6356	0.6425
0.1183	0.6513	0.5841	0.3132	0.9297	0.2688	0.4968	0.6058
0.3752	0.1703	0.3342	0.9950	0.2565	0.5974	0.2996	0.1190
0.8385	0.5028	0.3399	0.7348	0.8514	0.0365	0.3516	0.2659
0.3137	0.6962	0.1467	0.9515	0.7678	0.0470	0.0997	0.1320
0.0389	0.7888	0.7604	0.0432	0.1046	0.2107	0.0410	0.7398
0.6203	0.5192	0.1907	0.0816	0.4043	0.3911	0.7075	0.0028
0.3379	0.3839	0.4994	0.3116	0.3627	0.6780	0.8200	0.1826
0.5318	0.9266	0.4122	0.3772	0.1215	0.0306	0.7219	0.3187
0.1247	0.3259	0.3539	0.0382	0.9803	0.0397	0.7015	0.5763
0.0981	0.2007	0.7032	0.9989	0.6360	0.7085	0.8540	0.5358
0.0648	0.5269	0.4576	0.0454	0.4749	0.1590	0.3062	0.1927
0.1409	0.4222	0.3948	0.9645	0.6387	0.1261	0.9620	0.0462

Table AIII.1   1000 random numbers from 0 to 1 (cont.)

0.0614	0.3921	0.2111	0.0273	0.6874	0.0005	0.8702	0.6638
0.6973	0.2076	0.3828	0.1218	0.9518	0.5770	0.8490	0.3943
0.6461	0.6766	0.9159	0.6758	0.2377	0.8222	0.7635	0.7908
0.4431	0.3997	0.4895	0.0600	0.6586	0.2365	0.4314	0.8072
0.2381	0.7725	0.5084	0.8167	0.1828	0.0569	0.0129	0.1661
0.9499	0.7031	0.5672	0.2165	0.4620	0.7649	0.7255	0.8259
0.5778	0.3063	0.6536	0.9944	0.4970	0.0584	0.3568	0.7438
0.5588	0.1789	0.3138	0.7729	0.9800	0.9716	0.8690	0.8643
0.8993	0.4146	0.6216	0.4989	0.5803	0.6465	0.6294	0.7115
0.1922	0.9298	0.1822	0.6644	0.9524	0.3656	0.8779	0.7393
0.3379	0.8527	0.1043	0.3695	0.0588	0.8149	0.0324	0.1917
0.3975	0.6095	0.3722	0.7921	0.3267	0.1556	0.8578	0.2357
0.2635	0.5894	0.5026	0.4550	0.4720	0.1893	0.0308	0.4761
0.6090	0.8069	0.7402	0.8534	0.0036	0.3411	0.4176	0.2126
0.5046	0.3296	0.9629	0.9723	0.3057	0.6889	0.3207	0.1690
0.6864	0.2341	0.8566	0.1792	0.4122	0.0537	0.1500	0.5088
0.6708	0.7015	0.3896	0.4546	0.9458	0.7780	0.2261	0.7747
0.5091	0.5117	0.0624	0.9659	0.8695	0.3082	0.7528	0.0909
0.6178	0.3804	0.6908	0.1511	0.8540	0.6582	0.1398	0.7186
0.9481	0.4950	0.5676	0.3703	0.5378	0.3759	0.9840	0.4821
0.0230	0.3489	0.4001	0.8195	0.6568	0.7889	0.2681	0.2730
0.7363	0.5389	0.0133	0.2268	0.9699	0.3023	0.1212	0.6522
0.0993	0.4240	0.1393	0.6443	0.4266	0.2613	0.6562	0.8307
0.6990	0.5053	0.3248	0.7347	0.5635	0.4143	0.7973	0.9607
0.8614	0.4821	0.6950	0.4954	0.2531	0.7986	0.7323	0.1764
0.1507	0.5390	0.0998	0.1193	0.8367	0.1281	0.9030	0.8821
0.3288	0.3063	0.9083	0.7982	0.4531	0.1069	0.0498	0.3222
0.7832	0.3883	0.2298	0.7697	0.5826	0.1296	0.1918	0.2640
0.8148	0.0511	0.0553	0.6050	0.6665	0.7856	0.4468	0.3252
0.9495	0.6813	0.7001	0.1813	0.1231	0.5973	0.3411	0.8506
0.8420	0.0975	0.2229	0.5465	0.7489	0.0337	0.3961	0.5036
0.5089	0.4609	0.9633	0.6181	0.3741	0.8709	0.1698	0.4152
0.8548	0.1544	0.8301	0.9389	0.7664	0.5868	0.5947	0.9942
0.3324	0.0328	0.4804	0.9699	0.8740	0.0971	0.6262	0.6038

Table AIII.1 1000 random numbers from 0 to 1 (cont.)

0.8311	0.7386	0.3144	0.6620	0.2551	0.9304	0.5958	0.7693
0.1988	0.3582	0.5110	0.5026	0.4609	0.5222	0.2427	0.1150
0.1197	0.6459	0.0460	0.2834	0.7599	0.3732	0.5821	0.5995
0.9201	0.2320	0.3967	0.8042	0.5595	0.3466	0.4532	0.1495
0.8912	0.8219	0.5156	0.7422	0.3549	0.6961	0.4244	0.4253
0.1574	0.2107	0.2132	0.9118	0.7312	0.0803	0.2350	0.8643
0.5746	0.8711	0.5772	0.4445	0.6988	0.8400	0.2539	0.9453
0.0222	0.8208	0.9436	0.4136	0.2159	0.6660	0.4097	0.1204
0.0322	0.1602	0.8644	0.5753	0.9623	0.9110	0.9706	0.7809
0.1789	0.4832	0.6947	0.9608	0.1526	0.7107	0.5149	0.4749
0.8216	0.8724	0.7923	0.3492	0.6679	0.6719	0.6129	0.8891
0.1030	0.2197	0.1204	0.0305	0.5269	0.7606	0.1658	0.2936
0.6447	0.5800	0.3497	0.5190	0.5248	0.9854	0.5345	0.1202
0.3520	0.4562	0.8533	0.6140	0.6343	0.4687	0.5039	0.2005
0.6756	0.8372	0.5118	0.3571	0.0272	0.4183	0.0598	0.4212
0.1027	0.6699	0.5659	0.1363	0.3861	0.2237	0.0914	0.1153
0.1214	0.3845	0.8356	0.5619	0.9566	0.4510	0.2685	0.1914
0.8481	0.1510	0.4478	0.0571	0.4452	0.5447	0.6476	0.1760
0.4713	0.4062	0.1088	0.8944	0.1906	0.8993	0.2235	0.2823
0.0274	0.9728	0.7740	0.7520	0.5859	0.5672	0.7030	0.0416
0.5620	0.9396	0.5733	0.9635	0.2909	0.5111	0.8936	0.0038
0.6863	0.6889	0.3160	0.6812	0.3666	0.2688	0.7777	0.3953
0.4015	0.1611	0.8935	0.4905	0.8426	0.0230	0.2702	0.7094
0.3441	0.7391	0.6805	0.3313	0.0377	0.5288	0.8905	0.9740
0.5943	0.1807	0.1034	0.3676	0.2840	0.4029	0.7789	0.7057
0.7134	0.5990	0.4906	0.8852	0.8651	0.3197	0.8611	0.5856
0.3774	0.9146	0.0559	0.4561	0.1054	0.7134	0.8588	0.9297
0.9769	0.2236	0.5949	0.1089	0.8212	0.9666	0.7311	0.5052
0.1879	0.9701	0.6788	0.9791	0.8812	0.3184	0.9321	0.6815
0.4805	0.8146	0.0537	0.2141	0.0507	0.4943	0.2034	0.7287
0.6119	0.9841	0.4415	0.9273	0.7886	0.2068	0.6477	0.3388
0.0393	0.0489	0.6208	0.3309	0.1215	0.8672	0.9402	0.5593
0.5764	0.7096	0.0957	0.0579	0.0665	0.7751	0.2146	0.9081
0.0342	0.5974	0.9732	0.2892	0.2877	0.4920	0.1871	0.8618

Table AIII.1 1000 random numbers from 0 to 1 (cont.)

0.2071	0.7680	0.3068	0.5507	0.8490	0.7790	0.0092	0.9105
0.9752	0.4796	0.9963	0.4259	0.1921	0.6855	0.5749	0.5322
0.4157	0.5249	0.4410	0.7148	0.2178	0.4495	0.4241	0.8404
0.9686	0.0530	0.3452	0.9872	0.7481	0.6526	0.0748	0.8863
0.3588	0.5104	0.8449	0.5823	0.2146	0.1905	0.0106	0.8136
0.6133	0.4629	0.4962	0.4813	0.6105	0.2307	0.7349	0.0655
0.7831	0.0964	0.2129	0.8325	0.1896	0.1396	0.4171	0.6205
0.8250	0.0834	0.7948	0.4713	0.1797	0.4998	0.7562	0.0950
0.0503	0.1323	0.7946	0.7029	0.8900	0.1130	0.0046	0.0527
0.1190	0.3372	0.3816	0.8090	0.7792	0.4187	0.1932	0.7318
0.5578	0.0176	0.4983	0.9904	0.0190	0.3527	0.6703	0.2160
0.3310	0.1010	0.4120	0.1417	0.1427	0.2829	0.0761	0.8826
0.2270	0.8876	0.0901	0.8966	0.8685	0.7642	0.8832	0.9855
0.1933	0.9753	0.6777	0.3284	0.9558	0.7806	0.0528	0.0021
0.8168	0.4293	0.0075	0.9530	0.4237	0.3192	0.1024	0.1114
0.3860	0.3739	0.6006	0.0807	0.2597	0.9596	0.9319	0.7433
0.2576	0.3081	0.3683	0.9334	0.7564	0.5362	0.5170	0.4062
0.7653	0.8895	0.6684	0.3844	0.4876	0.2885	0.3242	0.0527
0.6862	0.7437	0.1962	0.6871	0.4455	0.1947	0.5027	0.4567
0.5604	0.2390	0.1577	0.6243	0.9104	0.9464	0.7771	0.2088
0.1321	0.3796	0.9836	0.5497	0.8878	0.0369	0.4062	0.2179
0.8303	0.4641	0.5111	0.5687	0.2380	0.4704	0.4228	0.5557
0.8079	0.5276	0.3555	0.7448	0.8160	0.4190	0.2636	0.4391
0.0897	0.3790	0.2979	0.7238	0.5371	0.4016	0.2408	0.9928
0.9592	0.1307	0.8048	0.2769	0.8930	0.2797	0.8596	0.4973
0.0790	0.9936	0.4660	0.3537	0.1799	0.6866	0.5731	0.2357
0.0850	0.1267	0.8106	0.8304	0.0362	0.6905	0.8594	0.6849
0.6099	0.7387	0.2769	0.7471	0.7851	0.9758	0.1695	0.7887
0.3970	0.3466	0.3917	0.0763	0.9484	0.3954	0.6780	0.8061
0.3532	0.8538	0.5508	0.0129	0.4960	0.6811	0.3646	0.0076
0.2693	0.7463	0.5141	0.4259	0.2930	0.8671	0.1009	0.6806
0.1896	0.1675	0.4605	0.9575	0.1980	0.1819	0.5230	0.9841
0.3155	0.0325	0.3460	0.5803	0.9713	0.1152	0.7375	0.5194
0.8478	0.2101	0.7787	0.3185	0.9690	0.6950	0.9906	0.9313
0.6125	0.7225	0.8982	0.8328	0.6478	0.9582	0.0591	0.9995

References

Altman, D.G. (1991) *Practical statistics for medical research.* Chapman and Hall.

Bell, J. (1993) *Doing your research project.* Open University Press, Buckingham.

British Medical Journal (editorial) (1999) 'Can it work? Does it work? Is it worth it? *BMJ* 319, 652–3.

Cryer, P. (1996) *The research student's guide to success.* Open University Press, Buckingham.

Dey, I. (1993) *Qualitative data analysis.* Routledge, London.

Gore, S.M. and Altman, D.G. (1982) *Statistics in practice.* British Medical Association, London.

Kreuger, R.A. (1994) *Focus groups: A practical guide for applied research.* Sage Publications, London.

Miles, M.B. and Huberman, A.M. (1994) *Qualitative data analysis.* Sage Publications, Thousand Oaks.

Robson, C. (1993) *Real world research.* Blackwell, Oxford.

Silverman, D. (1993) *Interpreting qualitative data.* Sage Publications, London.

Strauss, A. and Corbin, J. (1990) *Basics of qualitative research.* Sage Publications, Newbury Park.

Turnbull, L., Wood, N. and Kester, G. (1998) 'Controlled trial of the subjective patient benefits of walking to the operating theatre'. *International Journal of Clinical Practice*, Vol 52 No 2, 81–83.

Wood, N., Wilkinson, C. and Kumar, A. (1997) 'Do the homeless get a fair deal from general practitioners?' *Journal of the Royal Society of Health.* Vol 117, 292–297.

Index